The Sociology of Fun

Ben Fincham

The Sociology of Fun

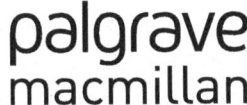

Ben Fincham
Department of Sociology
University of Sussex
Brighton, UK

ISBN 978-0-230-35857-7   ISBN 978-1-137-31579-3 (eBook)
DOI 10.1057/978-1-137-31579-3

Library of Congress Control Number: 2016945178

© The Editor(s) (if applicable) and The Author(s) 2016
The author(s) has/have asserted their right(s) to be identified as the author(s) of this work in accordance with the Copyright, Designs and Patents Act 1988.
This work is subject to copyright. All rights are solely and exclusively licensed by the Publisher, whether the whole or part of the material is concerned, specifically the rights of translation, reprinting, reuse of illustrations, recitation, broadcasting, reproduction on microfilms or in any other physical way, and transmission or information storage and retrieval, electronic adaptation, computer software, or by similar or dissimilar methodology now known or hereafter developed.
The use of general descriptive names, registered names, trademarks, service marks, etc. in this publication does not imply, even in the absence of a specific statement, that such names are exempt from the relevant protective laws and regulations and therefore free for general use.
The publisher, the authors and the editors are safe to assume that the advice and information in this book are believed to be true and accurate at the date of publication. Neither the publisher nor the authors or the editors give a warranty, express or implied, with respect to the material contained herein or for any errors or omissions that may have been made.

Cover illustration: © Everyright Images/Alamy Stock Photo

Printed on acid-free paper

This Palgrave Macmillan imprint is published by Springer Nature
The registered company is Macmillan Publishers Ltd. London

*For my children Nancy and Joshua
and my grandmother Betty Hutchings.
This was her idea really.*

Acknowledgements

My thanks go to the first cohort of students that took the Third Year Undergraduate Course, 'A Sociology of Fun', in the Department of Sociology at the University of Sussex in the spring of 2014. They are an inspirational group of people who gave themselves wholeheartedly to the study of fun. So, thanks and credit to Laurie Amar, Sophie Anscombe, Charlene Aure, Ashley Barnes, Megan Bond, Rhyanna Coleman, Jess Di Simone, Geraint Harries, Zsuzsa Holmes, Rosie Hyam, Jennie Leighton, Juliette Martin Useo, Ella Matthews, Jess Midgely, Becky Reynolds, Amy Sarjeant, Beth White and Lainey White.

Thanks must also go to the 201 people that took part in the 'fun' survey.

I would like to thank people working at the Salvage Café in Hove in the spring and summer of 2015, where much of this book was written. In particular, I would like to say thank you to Matthew English, Tazz Khan, Lauren Joy Kennett, Holly Macve and Joshua Taylor who were patient in the face of what must have seemed like some weird questions at times.

I would like to thank Palgrave Macmillan publishers, especially Philippa Grand, Beth O'Leary, Harriet Barker and Amelia Derkatsch for their support and encouragement during the production of this book.

Finally, I would like to thank my family. My mum and dad, Deborah and Barry, who provided the perfect backdrop for my fun growing up—I realise how lucky I am that they are my parents. I want to thank my brother, Joe—who probably does not know how prominently he features in my stories of fun throughout my life. Now my partner, Bree, is providing the perfect backdrop for my and my children's fun—which is as important to me as anything. Thank you, Bree.

Contents

1	Introduction	1
2	Theorising Fun	27
3	Fun and Games: Childhood	47
4	Fun and Frivolity: Adulthood	83
5	Fun at Work	121
6	Phenomenal Fun	155
7	Fun and Recollection	183
8	Conclusions	197
Bibliography		207
Index		209

List of Figures

Fig. 2.1	Schema of fun	40
Fig. 4.1	Average personal wellbeing by age group UK 2012–13	91

1

Introduction

Towards a Sociology of Fun

Fun is taken for granted. In everyday talk people use the term anticipating that others will know what they mean when they describe something as fun. In fact it is so taken for granted that outside of dictionary definitions there is very little in the way of explanations for what fun is and how to discern it from other social experiences. What we know is that sometimes we have it and sometimes we don't, one person's idea of it is not necessarily another's and having too much of it is often frowned upon. Much of the literature that is used in this book refers to fun as rooted in activities presumed to be fun—'camping and water-based activities' are 'popular and fun' according to a study of 'rural family fun' (Churchill et al. 2007: 282)[1]—or conflates fun with things like play (Yee 2006; Churchill et al. 2007; Kelty et al. 2008), happiness (Cameron 1972; Jackson 2000; Sumnall et al. 2010), leisure (Scanlan and Simons 1992; Bengoechea et al. 2004; MacPhail et al. 2008) or deviance (Riemer 1981; Redmon 2003; Keppens and Spruyt 2015). Whilst it is the case that all of these

---

[1] Clearly this will be a moot point for those that hate camping.

areas may contain elements that people would describe as fun, there is precious little in the way of theorising or describing what it is. Fun pertains to other areas of life but is rarely viewed as a defining feature of it. The most pertinent example of this is found in the recent interest in issues of happiness and well-being. Opinions and expertise on happiness emanate from a wide array of academic disciplinary backgrounds. People working in psychology, psychiatry, economics, social policy, health studies, philosophy, geography and youth studies—to name a few—have been applying themselves to understanding what constitutes happiness, its relationship to well-being, how to measure it and importantly how to instil a sense of it in individuals and populations (Rodriguez et al. 2011; Bok 2010; Veenhoven 2009; Waite et al. 2009; Diener and Biswas-Diener 2008). At the same time as the world economic recession of 2008–2009 reverberated through economies several national governments became interested in measures of happiness in populations. In the UK the government decided to conduct a survey through the Office for National Statistics to assess how 'happy' the British population was in 2011 (Directgov 2010). The intention of officially monitoring happiness was to steer government social policy (Stratton 2010). Elsewhere, the governments of France and Canada developed national happiness measures at the same time as the UK (Stratton 2010). The discussions about happiness and well-being were generally centred on a few core themes, the most prominent being wealth and income, job satisfaction, feelings of community, relationships with friends and family, environment, cultural activities, health and education (Directgov 2010). The thinking is that if you can get a sense of these facets of a person's life as successful or unsuccessful, attained or unattained, then you should be able to infer levels of happiness. However, the point for this book is not to dwell on the obvious difficulties in defining and then measuring something subjective like levels of happiness—or whether it is a worthwhile pursuit or not—but to note that there has been an important omission from almost all discussions about what makes people happy—namely, *fun*. The absence of fun perhaps relates to the conflation of happiness with well-being where fun is peripheral to the more weighty matters of physical health or economic security—but when considered alongside happiness, this absence is odd. During two particular studies I have been involved with, one looking at informal labour markets and the other into the relationship between mental health and work, the importance of fun to people became apparent. In interviews when asked what made them happy—particularly at work—many participants identified having fun as a fundamental reason for being happy. Obviously, this is not a novel observation, as Donald Roy points out in *Banana Time* several commentators in the 1950s had made similar points. As an interviewee in work on assembly line workers by Walker and Guest said, 'We have a lot of fun and talk all the time... if it weren't for the talking and fooling you'd go nuts' (Roy 1959: 158). The role of fun for making situations at worst tolerable and at best enjoyable is clear—which is what makes the omission of fun as an object of serious study all the more perplexing. There is a general absence of any engagement with fun as a central feature of happiness; rather, fun is a by-product of activities that are supposed to make us happy. This book is an attempt primarily to acknowledge the central role fun plays in our lives and also to develop a sociological approach to fun.

By way of an introduction to fun and sociology, this chapter establishes the parameters within which the rest of the book operates. Here a sociological definition of fun is, very broadly, outlined. There is a description of how fun has been conceptualised by academics historically—with specific reference to the 1950s literature on 'fun morality'. There is an account of references to fun outside of sociology and many of these will be picked up in further chapters. Important for a sociological definition are the ways in which fun operates differently in various contexts—work, family, education, leisure, and so on—and this contextual aspect is highlighted here. It is also in the introduction that the distinctiveness of fun as performing specific social functions—and its relationship to power—is introduced. After the historical view, further debates that the book engages with are outlined. More generally, the book questions the 'taken for granted' nature of references to fun. Do people mean the same things when they talk about 'having fun'? Why is one person's idea of fun different from somebody else's? The relationship between fun, happiness and well-being is also addressed. This is the first book that explicitly sets out a 'sociology of fun'. As such it is an exploration of the different ways that fun features in everyday life and how sociology can bring something distinctive to that analysis.

The Importance of Fun

As I have indicated, the idea for a concerted study of fun emerged during 2010–2011. Carl Walker and I had just published a book called *Work and the Mental Health Crisis in Britain* (Walker and Fincham 2011) and it was also the period in which the UK government, under the premiership of David Cameron, was developing the 'National Wellbeing Programme'. This initiative had disappeared from public consciousness fairly soon after an initial flurry of interest—but the aim, according to the Office for National Statistics, was to 'produce accepted and trusted measures of the well-being of the nation' (Office for National Statistics 2011). They went on to broadly define well-being and talk about why it was important to try and measure it:

> Well-being put simply is about 'how we are doing' as individuals, as communities and as a nation and how sustainable this is for the future. Measuring National Well-being is about looking at 'GDP and beyond'. (Office for National Statistics 2011)

It is worth noting that the government became interested in measuring well-being in the depths of the worst economic recession since the 1930s. A cynic might suggest that this interest was inspired by a government trying to suggest that GDP is not the best way to rate the success of any given society at a time when the economy was going from bad to worse. This view was hardly undermined by the disappearance of governmental concern in measuring well-being during the economic recovery. However, my interest was piqued by what I had noticed in the study of mental health and work and a significant absence in the well-being index survey. During the study of the relationship between work, employment and workers' feelings of mental well-being, an interesting dichotomy emerged in interviews in relation to the idea of fun. On the one hand, interviewees talked about how important it was to have fun whilst at work and that it not only signalled good relationships between colleagues but was also a key factor for continued healthy engagement with work. On the other hand, when describing instances of fun, people represented it as frivolous, unimportant in relation to other aspects of being at work. It seemed to be something to be a bit embarrassed about (Walker and Fincham 2011). It was also clear that the way people were framing fun in their own lives was distinct, but related to, ideas of happiness.

In the ONS survey there was no mention of fun at all. There was no attempt to assess the role fun played in a person's sense of well-being. In fact I could not find specific mentions of fun in any of the many well-being indexes being developed at the time (Canadian Index of Wellbeing 2015; Office for National Statistics 2015; OECD 2015; The State of the USA 2015). The implication was that well-being is predicated on certain aspects of life, but fun is not one of them.

These two trains of thought led to a very simple existential question. What would a life without any fun be like? Just asking the question summons up a terribly bleak scenario. If the absence of fun is so bad, then it must be important. If you think through the implications of the question, and where an absence of fun impacts, it is squarely in the realms of happiness and well-being—it is a very bad thing to have no fun.

In terms of well-being and happiness people are happier than they would otherwise be if they have fun.

It became apparent quite early on that fun is complicated. It is a multi-dimensional, multifunctional social phenomenon. It defines experiences, characterises people, embellishes memories; it feeds moments with positivity, establishes the conditions for good relationships; it draws distinctions between good and bad times and it enhances life. It is curiously ambiguous—we know when we are having it, but struggle to define it.

Do We Know What Fun Is?

As is often the case, in books like this dictionary definitions are only useful in as much as they provide a starting point but little else. The *Oxford English Dictionary* (*OED*) describes fun as 'diversion, amusement, sport; also, boisterous jocularity or gaiety, drollery. Also, a source or cause of amusement or pleasure' (Oxford English Dictionary Online 2011). This clearly does not encompass our experience of fun. The semantics of experiences are difficult, and as an approximation dictionary definitions are always reductive—but for something as profound and significant as fun, the *OED* inevitably lacks depth. My disquiet about this definition is in part because of the etymology of the word *fun*. Its meaning has diversified over the centuries from describing cheating in the seventeenth century to a pejorative description of low wit or mockery in the nineteenth century to its modern meaning, associating fun with 'exciting goings on' (Blythe and Hassenzahl 2004: 92). The history of the word *fun* is suffused social class, judgement and transgression. Blythe and Hassenzahl give a particularly illuminating and concise explanation of the role of the industrial revolution in shaping contemporary notions of fun. They explain that in the routinisation and mechanisation of work the boundaries between work and leisure—or not being at work—became clear, but more importantly, the processes of rationalisation *in* work leads to the development of fun as a mode of resistance to routine and regimentation. This, and an association of a lack of middle- or upper-class sophistication with fun, made it a working class, subversive activity. To a certain extent this can still be seen today, particularly in the rhetoric of 'taking the piss' or 'having a laugh'. As will be explored later in the book, there is often a transgressive or subversive element to the ways in which we have fun—and this is still often associated with a lack of sophistication. This chequered past echoes in contemporary settings, and this in turn needs to be factored in to any account of what fun is today. These echoes do not necessarily have to refer to industrialisation and class specifically, but make sense of the outside or transgressive element that is often a component of fun. As will be addressed later, the trivialisation or marginalisation of fun—when it is so important to feeling good—may have closer ties to social control and productivity than we care to imagine.

Despite sporadic interest in fun in a variety of contexts, there has never been a sustained attempt to pin down what is meant by fun. There are a number of reasons as to why this might be. For example, Goffman suggests in *Encounters*:

> Because serious activity need not justify itself in terms of the fun it provides, we have neglected to develop an analytical view of fun and an appreciation of the light fun throws on interaction in general. (Goffman 1961: 17)

Blythe and Hassenzahl (2004) are rare for their attempt to systematically address how to theorise fun and whilst there are many references to it in various places, there is rarely any attempt to explain what the phenomenon is. Rather, it is up to the reader or listener to fill in the gaps by inferring fun from references to other things—happiness, laughter or whatever. So, whilst many people refer to fun, few try to pin down what they or—in the case of empirical research—their participants/informants mean when they talk about it. As I say, these oblique references mean that we have to infer from the points of reference used by writers when they talk about fun.

For example, the relationship between leisure, culture and consumption gives clues as a hegemonic construct of fun through capitalist provision of leisure spaces/activities and the development of leisure industries. Whilst not directly addressing fun they, nonetheless, often called upon fun as the motivation for the consumption of particular leisure activities and/or products. The relationship between sporting activities and fun, particularly when encouraging youth participation, predominates references to fun and leisure (Fine 1989; Seefeldt et al 1993; Siegenthalter and Gonzalez 1997; Jackson 2000; Strean and Holt 2000; Bengoechea et al 2004; Macphail et al 2008). Generally the term 'fun' is used quite unreflexively and an assumption is made that we all know what it means, even when we acknowledge that it means different things to different people. For example, Bengoechea et al. (2004) correctly state that fun has different meanings depending on perspective and context. In their study of fun in youth sport, Bengoechea et al. first point out that fun and enjoyment are distinct yet related (Bengoechea et al. 2004: 198) and then immediately say that 'for research purposes fun and enjoyment should be considered synonymous because "fun" is the term that children commonly use to refer to enjoyable experiences' (198). Later in the same paper, a section is dedicated to discerning 'different meanings in fun' (204)—differences observed in the testimonies of sports coaches are reduced to 'achievement and non-achievement dimensions of the experience of fun' (204), the former accentuating winning or striving to win being associated with fun and the latter concentrating more on 'pleasure and avoiding pain' (206). What is interesting in this example is the difficulty the authors have in specifying what the phenomenon being reported to them consists of.

For a start, the interviewees are all adult coaches and not children, so the initial conflation of fun and enjoyment is curious—unless the authors imagine that adults use the terms interchangeably also. A telling part of the paper that highlights the problem for many commentators in this field of study is the association of fun with wasting time fecklessness but the understanding that fun is what many people want to have. Once again in the Bengoechea et al. example:

> A comment by Carla, a rowing coach (boys and girls, 14–18) illustrated potential negative connotations of fun when depicted as non-achievement, non-performance aspect of sport: 'like I don't like the word "fun" because it implies, you know, fooling around, and carefree, and not paying attention.' Scanlon and colleagues (Scanlon and Simons 1992; Scanlon et al. 1993) have noted that the enjoyment construct suffers from a pre-conceived notion of frivolity or what they refer to as the 'pizza parlor phenomenon'. (Bengoechea et al. 2004: 205)

The conflation of fun and enjoyment in studies of sport is common (MacPhail et al. 2008; Bengoechea et al 2004; Scanlan and Simons 1992) but so is the observation that fun is something that is distinct and often distracting. Strean and Holt suggest that fun should be considered a 'subset' of enjoyment, so, whilst one could experience enjoyment and not describe it as fun, fun is always enjoyable. Their conclusion comes from the persistent idea in sports studies of 'positive affective' responses to sport (Strean and Holt 2000: 85). It is difficult to disagree with the simple assertion that fun is always enjoyable, but this is something that I will return to later in the book—as with much of fun it is not that straightforward.

In the introduction to his excellent edited collection *For Fun and Profit*, Richard Butsch summarises key debates in studies of leisure. Of particular interest is the argument that developed between those that saw the provision of officially sanctioned leisure activities for the 'working classes'— parks, playhouses, bars, and so on—as social control in action and those that concentrated on the ways in which these activities or spaces were subverted by those for whom they were supposed to be provided (Butsch 1990: 6–7). Once again, fun as a form of resistance comes into focus.

Rather than being something benign and pleasurable it becomes active, subversive and pleasurable, attempts to control the fun of others becomes a site of classed contestation.[2] This disruptive and uncomfortable aspect of fun may be partly responsible for the lack of serious consideration it is given. In terms of class war there are many other elements of resistance that Marxists have preferred to concentrate on—none of them much fun. I suppose the conflict model doesn't foster the idea that something as apparently harmless as fun could actually be part of some rhetoric of resistance. Interestingly, it is from the school of Symbolic Interactionism that the subversive nature of fun in industrial settings is most obviously described (Roy 1959).

Obviously conceptual conflation is not just reserved for fun. When examining the literature on happiness and well-being, it soon becomes apparent that these terms are used interchangeably as though they are the same thing (e.g., Veenhoven 1991; Graham 2012; Brülde 2015). This is, of course, not the case. When considering physical health in relation to well-being, or economic security in relation to well-being, for example, the multifaceted nature of the term is apparent. As even the UK well-being index implies, there is more to well-being than happiness. Not just that but general well-being might be considered low for a person but they might feel relatively happy. This relational aspect of happiness causes problems for attempts to measure it, and also to work out how integral it is to well-being. For many I suspect it is a matter of priorities. Some people would think that physical health and healthy finances are at least as important as feeling happy (whatever that means) or that happiness is not really possible without those things being well. Others would think that happiness is so contextually bound that it is not possible to fit it into a schema of overall well-being—and that it is not just dependent on static features of life like income or physical health. However, an implication of conflating happiness and well-being is that it further excludes fun from being considered an important feature of social life. It is more a positive by-product of the more important things—happiness and/or well-being.

---

[2] This is perhaps an echo of things like the tradition of the 'Lord of Misrule' in the UK—a practice Henry VIII tried to ban in 1541 with limited success.

By the time people are talking about well-being, fun has already been folded into happiness as a component of it, rather than a discrete element of social life that is related to it.

Fun, Morality and Identity

Whilst fun is something that is experienced, it also has a strong discursive element. As is indicated in the commentary on the etymology of the word, there has been a classed side to fun, and an association with crassness or fecklessness—and today with wasting time or not doing the serious important stuff. At the same time, it is something that we crave and want to be associated with. Martha Wolfenstein's idea of 'fun morality' (Wolfenstein 1951) has been very important to my own thinking about fun. For her there was a transformation in attitudes to having fun provoked largely as a response to changes brought about by the Second World War and a transformation in attitudes to play. Before the war according to Wolfenstein both play and fun carried negative connotations. Fun was frivolous and base, unsophisticated and crude, play was associated with 'unhealthy excitement and nervous debilitation'. Throughout the 1940s, in the USA, both fun and play were reimagined. For the post-war generation of youngsters play was about 'muscular development, necessary exercise, strength, and control' (Wolfenstein 1951, 20). Similarly, fun was transformed from being something to be avoided to being obligatory. It was something to be had and displayed in conjunction with play:

> As the mother is urged to make play an aspect of every activity, play assumes a new obligatory quality... Thus it is now not adequate for the mother to perform efficiently the necessary routines for her baby; she must also see that these are fun for both of them... Play, having ceased to be wicked, having become harmless and good becomes now a duty (Wolfenstein 1951, 20)

According to Wolfenstein the transformation of play and fun had a profound effect on the ways in which people in the USA came to see a demonstration of having fun as integral to how people perceived each other. The aspiration or pressure was to be known as a fun gal or a fun guy and if this were the case it was an example of a life being well lived. As the quote suggests this was most acutely felt by mothers of young children. The moral aspect of fun highlighted by Wolfenstein has been a consistent theme relating to it. It was during a lecture that I was delivering to undergraduates that I started to think about the representation of fun identities online. The issues arising from identity management and the consequences of mismanaged online representations are documented (Thomas 2007; Young 2013), and it strikes me that a similar process of identity management is going on within social media where the imperative to appear a particular way—in relation to fun—is strong. People, particularly young people, tend to post images of themselves having fun on holiday, fun in the bar, fun on the beach, fun with friends, fun by themselves, fun in the shops, fun in the café and fun everywhere. The same pressure, described by Wolfenstein in the 1950s, is alive and kicking here in the twenty-first century. Nobody has *that* much fun, but to represent ourselves as either not having much fun, or worse, not much fun ourselves, is a risky strategy. In conversations with colleagues and friends it has become clear that there are implications to not being seen as much fun. In fact ongoing research by Tamsin Hinton-Smith and myself suggests that a 'not much fun' identity can have serious consequences for career progression in certain employment sectors, particularly for women (Hinton-Smith and Fincham 2016).

Fun and Power

An area that has been covered pretty well in studies of humour is that of power. Fun and humour are related, and the number of instances where either moments of humour or continuous humour, throughout an evening, for example, were cited by respondents to my survey was many. However, the importance of power in humour as highlighted by Michael Billig, for example, is not nearly so important for fun (Billig 2005). In Billig's account it is the maintenance of power inequalities that services much humour—particularly in relation to cruelty. This is not the case with fun according to Podilchak. For him there is an overt reference to relationships between people, rather than activities, that manifest as fun.

He suggests that fun is actually the materialisation of social conditions in which freedom and choice to adopt positive affective positions occurs. He suggests that 'fun is clearly established as a type of relationship construction rather than a specific activity' (Podilchak 1991: 135). Further, he says that

> [Fun] is a conscious restructuring if the social setting and its acceptance by interacting persons which produces an emotional reward, not strictly the intention to be playful. The intention has to be materialised, and the normative frame is the equality of interacting members. (Podilchak 1991: 136)

For him fun can only properly occur when power differentials and hierarchies are ignored or not present:

> The feelings of fun only emerge in this social bond and require an equality condition among members. I propose that the interactants have temporarily deconstructed their biographical and social inequalities. The establishment of a sharing friendship, where the 'fun is spread' is identified. Fun only lasts as long as these inequality and power differentials are negated ... Fun is deemed less serious only because the equality mechanism in 'human-ness' challenges the ideological justification of the ideological justification of the differentiated hierarchical social condition. (Podilchak 1991: 145)

Podilchak highlights the persistent issue of the subjective experience of fun on the one hand and a structural determination on the other. The hierarchies to which he refers are artefacts of structure that are invested in biographies. For him the conditions for fun only arise when these biographical and social inequalities have been flattened out, as opposed to humour where power differentials are perpetuated or accentuated.

Power is clearly important to understanding social contexts and, as Podilchak suggests, fun is a phenomena born out of relationships in contexts. The extent to which power in fun can be so absolutely understood, as is implied by Podilchak, is debatable. There are situations where fun is described because of the maintenance of power differentials, or where power is played with—not simply a negation of inequity. This is the case with more submissive forms of fun in situations where the excitement is accentuated by a ceding of power.

Contexts of Fun

Another major theme for this book is that fun is contextual—there are social circumstances that come about or are created that determine the sorts of fun that we have. These contexts are structurally and culturally bound—even when it is the most intimate and personal sort of fun. Our orientation to experiences is formed before the experience itself; in this respect, our reaction to experiences either supports or confounds the cultural and social expectations that we have of them—to echo Becker's 'On Becoming a Marijuana User' (Becker 1963), 'drugs are bad, but to my surprise I really enjoyed that E you gave me', 'drugs are bad and you trying to give me that E[3] spoiled my evening', 'drugs are bad, I had that E and I just felt very anxious all night' and 'drugs are good and that E you gave me really did the trick' (see Becker's 'Outsiders' (1963) for a much more full and nuanced explanation in relation to drugs, enjoyment, orientation and context). Despite fun being largely absent from accounts of experiences of aspects of everyday life, it is important to many of the contexts within which we operate socially. The following are all dealt with more specifically elsewhere in the book, but by way of introduction here are a few examples of clearly delineated areas of social life where fun is a significant component, but where it has been largely ignored. Any sustained consideration of these areas of social life in relation to fun provokes interesting questions.

Work

Despite recent attempts by a few major employers most people do not associate work with fun. In fact work has for many years has been represented as the counterweight to fun, which resides in other areas of activity, rather blithely referred to as 'life'. The discourse of work/life balance has intensified the characterisation of work as a place that distracts from pleasurable experiences—these happen elsewhere. Not only

---

[3] The recreational drug ecstasy.

is this an inaccurate portrayal of many people's experience of work, it also establishes expectations of work which, lo and behold, then become realised. As will be discussed, part of the problem for employers trying to encourage 'fun at work' is that fun is not something that can be stimulated on somebody else's terms. Even though it seems to be experienced in similar ways by similar people, the fun is owned by the individual. For my part, there are few things more galling at work than being told by a manager that I am going to have fun on a training day. This often means that an activity or event will have been designed to get me in the mood to share my thoughts, but in a fun way. My heart sinks at the prospect of this sort of managed fun. What happens in practice is that I do have fun not doing the thing that I am supposed to—being childish or slightly mutinous. The point is that unless we determine how and when we have fun, it doesn't seem to work. You cannot turn fun on and off like a tap. For most people time at work is organised according to somebody else's schedule. Most of us would not choose to spend time in the places that those that pay us demand. It is in this regimentation of time and task that fun finds its most common mischievous and transgressive expression. In the chapter on work and fun, there are examples where, for employees, fun is not doing what they are supposed to. However, this is just one part of the story of fun at work—and is easy to overstate. The most potent source of fun at work, as with everywhere else, is other people. Most people work with others and it is in these relationships that fun is created.

Family

The ideal type of a family involves stable relationships that are underpinned by love and concern for members. Each family evolves as members grow and in this evolution ways of doing are established—traditions and expectations. One of the most striking things in the data gathered for this book was the number of people for whom this ideal type appears to exist. Familial relations provided the context for an enormous amount of fun—especially in childhood. Whilst this might not be a surprise to many, I was anticipating far more in the way of stories about fun with peers and friends and also how families were an impediment to having fun—siblings getting in the way or parents not allowing their children to do what they wanted. I'm sure that if pushed in that direction people would have been able to tell me instances of this, but the overriding theme was that families were contexts where fun happened. Holidays were particularly prominent in the data and the association of fun with unusual or out of the ordinary goings-ons, to paraphrase Blythe and Hassenzahl, is clear. As with work, the family is a structural social phenomenon that, in all of its guises, provides a context within which things are experienced, and also similar to work our expectations of what happens in these structural contexts does not necessarily reflect what actually happens.

Education

Perhaps the most structurally bound space in which the majority of us spend time is education. Schools are all about rules and the enforcement of rules intensifies as we move through schooling. In early years teaching, in the UK, there is an emphasis on play and fun as key pedagogic tools. It is understood that young children learn best through active, fun learning. As young people progress through schooling, the emphasis moves inexorably away from fun towards serious scholarship. It is curious that whilst our brains are at their most elastic and gymnastic—in early childhood—we concede that play and fun are key instruments for learning, and as we then move through schooling, we sequester or marginalise fun until, by the time we are 16, fun is not what we are having in the classroom. Whilst we are learning to live by timetables and becoming trained for the workplace, we are also surreptitiously learning how and when to have subversive fun. The unbridled fun of early childhood has no particular rebellious qualities, but by the time we are teenagers it most certainly does. To a large extent, this is because the rules by which we are supposed to adhere are increasingly iterated and enforced. The sorts of things you can do as a child are not tolerated as we get older. Shouting or singing loudly in public, nudity whenever you feel like it, game playing, mess, frivolity are all components of early childhood that become increasingly regulated as we move through life. Bending the rules at school becomes increasingly a source of fun for many students as the opportunities for fun elsewhere at school diminish. School is also the place where a model for conducting friendships is established—but these friendships are visited and revisited almost every day. This repetition means that often it is the minutiae of everyday life that preoccupies talk between these groups of young people. It is little wonder then that repetition and a lack of seriousness underscores much of the peer interaction in schools. As will be reiterated throughout this book, the ways in which we socialise are key to understanding the fun that we have. So, in modern education systems we find the institutional structure that provides the template for how we, as adults, view having fun. For the sake of the institution fun is supposed to happen in designated periods of time—playtime—and the classroom is reserved for more serious and important pursuits. This is controlled by a timetable that determines how the day is supposed to look. Authority is to be respected regardless of whether it is sensibly administered or not. However, for those people going through school education fun is subversive—'cock a snook' at authority. In addition to fun at play or lunchtime, it is sometimes had at the times when it is not supposed to be, during lessons and in the classroom through mucking about, and it is all about yourself and others.

Leisure

Literature on leisure will be addressed in the next chapter. Studies of leisure and Veblen's 'Theory of the Leisure Class' (1899) informed thinking on this project from early on. The nominally dichotomous relationship between leisure and work means that it is an area where you expect to find fun. A modern conception of leisure is time spent away from laborious tasks, domestic, formally employed or whatever. It is in this time that we are supposed to enjoy, relax and perhaps have fun. This is all very well, but relaxing is difficult, and eking out time for enjoyment is fairly labour intensive—I am willing to concede that this might just be because I organise my life inefficiently—but fun is less dependent on these carved out tranches of time that things like relaxation or pleasurable things to do.

I think that the assumed intrinsic relationship between fun and leisure is less stable than we like to think. I am not suggesting that people do not enjoy leisure time nor that they don't have fun in leisure time, but they are not automatically related. As will be discussed in later chapters, particularly the one on *Phenomenal Fun*, whilst we might think we have fun doing certain things—because this is how we socially represent them—when you properly interrogate the experience people have of them, 'fun' is not the word that immediately springs to mind. Having sex I think is a good example of this—fun in popular discourse, but if you were to ask people in flagrante to describe what was happening to them, I doubt whether 'fun' would be high up the list—all sorts of other nice things perhaps, but not fun. The relationship of many things done in leisure time—pursuits—to commitment, learning, dedication, progression and often frustration—stands in contrast to the sorts of key defining features of fun for Blythe and Hassenzahl at least. In the next chapter I present a model of fun that I think allows for a more flexible interpretation of experiences than that offered by Blythe and Hassenzahl—but as a starting point for thinking about a model of fun their contribution has been, for me at least, invaluable.

Backdrops

The sorts of contexts that I have outlined above—work, family, education and leisure, for example—are general social contexts. As they are culturally and socially embedded, they provide the landscapes within which specific occasions of fun sit. These are the subjective experiences of fun that are unique to individuals, but these micro-contexts themselves are also backdrops to moments in time of fun. A way of illustrating this is to use stories of fun from different stages of life. When they are written down, the generalised nature of these completely unique experiences becomes clear. There is an inherent dichotomy in experiences of fun as on the one hand utterly unique to the person that is having/has had the fun and on the other hand the resonance and replicability of that fun to others' experiences.

For example, I can identify moments across my life, specific moments of fun, and these are set in contexts that I generally identify as spaces where fun happened. I am no writer of prose—as I am about to illustrate—but will try to show what I mean with three stories from three distinct periods of my own life:

As a child playing with my brother at the beach in Cornwall, where our grandmother lived, provides a backdrop where I understand fun to have happened. I can then summon up occasions where I had fun. When I was about ten years old, my grandmother led my parents, my brother and I on what seemed like a particularly hazardous descent onto the rocks next to Kenneggy Sands on the Cornish south coast. It was a beautiful sunny day, and when we finally made it onto the rocks, they were hot to the touch. The sea was a Mediterranean blue and the kelp beneath the water looked mysterious and inviting, rather than slightly menacing as it normally did to me. There was a deep wide fissure in the rocks where we had established ourselves and we were diving from a natural platform into this gap and out into the open sea. My grandmother and mother then decided we were going to swim beyond the cove. I had never swum in water that deep—it was thrilling and a little bit frightening—but they were there next to me. When we turned back, the view was stunning. We could see from Marazion past Rinsey Head to Porthleven. As we approached our rocky base the cliffs loomed above us—I hadn't noticed them on the way out—they were behind me. When we got out of the water, I lay on the warm rocks, drying almost instantly, and listened to a cassette on my Walkman that my aunt's boyfriend had made for me.

Another very specific backdrop is a band I was in when I was in my late teens with my friends Carl, Julian, Mikey and Johnny. We used to practise in a room in Carl's great-grandmother's bungalow—I should say she wasn't there at the time. One particular practice, we had been drinking alcohol in the afternoon and spent the rehearsal laughing and laughing as we murdered the songs that we had spent months rehearsing. We would compose ourselves after a bout of hysterics and Johnny would count us in—at which point one person would drunkenly mess up—whilst it doesn't sound funny now, at the time I thought it was the funniest thing that had ever happened.

More recently my children, Nancy and Joshua, provide a backdrop where I know fun happens—amongst other things. My partner, Bree, the children and I were at a music festival—the first that Joshua would remember. At the time both of the children loved a band called Public Service Broadcasting and they were on the bill. We had spent a fair amount of time at the festival, and though no fault of the kids, it had been quite tiring getting ourselves sorted out. We had something to eat and watched a couple of things on other stages and then made our way to the stage were Public Service Broadcasting were due to play. The band came on and the kids realised that these were the actual people off the CD! Dancing with them as they started to recognise the songs, having them on my shoulders shouting at the tops of their voices and watching them grinning from ear to ear was enormous fun.

I have hundreds of backdrops and thousands of instances and they coalesce into my way of experiencing fun. These are either relived in memory and narratives or deployed in the present to orient me towards experiences I am having or about to have. As a result, we tend to imagine that fun is a deeply subjective experience, and the thought that one person's idea of fun is not another's is a familiar one. As I have tried to illustrate with the stories above, our experiences and memories of it are distinctly ours. However, a major theme for this book is that fun is more uniformly experienced than we might imagine. That is not to say that it necessarily feels the same from person to person, but that it is culturally and socially mediated. A key assertion in this book is that fun is a social phenomenon. It is had with other people or in relation to other people, it is communicated in ways that make sense to others and it relates closely to our sense of social identity—who we think we are and who others think we are. I hope that my stories of fun strike a chord with you, because they sound like fun. You will recognise these experiences and relate them to experiences that you have had—and whilst the specifics may differ, I bet that thematically they are broadly similar to yours.

For this book I conducted a survey where people were asked a variety of questions about fun—memories from childhood, recent occasions of fun, questions about gender and the distinction between fun and happiness, amongst other things. The survey was conducted between April and

October 2014 using Bristol Online Survey. This online resource hosted the fun survey. Respondents followed a link to the survey and then completed it in their own time. The link was distributed via social networks and word of mouth. As a result, the sample is not representative; however, as the survey was qualitative in nature, representativeness was not a methodological intention. The survey was split into three sections. The first asked general demographic questions: age, gender, where the respondent lived, number of siblings and occupation. The second asked about experiences of fun: 'Tell me about an occasion in your childhood where you had fun (if you are still a younger person tell me about a time when you were even smaller)'; 'Tell me about a recent occasion where you had fun'; 'Do boys and girls have fun in the same way?'; 'Do you think women and men have fun differently?'; 'If you work (full or part time), how do you have fun at work?'. The third section asked about definitions of fun: 'Please try and describe to me what "having fun" feels like'; 'So... what is fun? How is it different from happiness or pleasure?'

There were 201 responses by the time the survey closed in October. The majority of respondents (79%) were between the ages of 20 and 50; 68% were women, 31% men, 1% trans and 2% other. A key feature of the demographic was the occupational profile. As the sampling method was essentially snowball and opportunistic, the sample is heavily biased towards middle-class occupations. Whilst social class and fun is an issue that is not addressed directly in this book, it does merit further interrogation.

For coding, in the analysis of the data, I tried to be inventive and wide in my codes. After the first round of coding of the 201 responses, I had over 100 codes; this increased after the second detailed run-through. However, when it came to grouping the codes thematically, it was much easier than I had anticipated with that many codes. There are, of course, a few codes that did not fit within the broader categories—in many ways, these are the most interesting stories. As will become apparent in all of the chapters involving data from the fun survey, there are crossovers all over the place between themes. As fun is relational it is to be expected that when people talk about it they talk in relational, comparative and integrative ways. There were very few occasions where what a person said fitted neatly into one category or, in terms of analysis, code.

One indication that there is something culturally significant about the testimonies is that they resonate so pertinently for others with a similar cultural vocabulary. Put simply, I recognised and enjoyed and think shared so many of the experiences or stories having grown up in the same place and time as many people that lent me their memories.

The survey only asked for single instances and also there were no follow-up questions so the chance for elucidation or increased individuality in the stories was not possible—still the variety in the responses to the question about a recent instance of fun (normally in adulthood apart from the children in the survey) and fun in childhood was marked. I will discuss why I think this apparent uniformity occurs a little later.

One of the reasons the results were so good to read was that the fun described by people was easy for me to identify with—and the glue that bound the narratives was that, at its heart, fun is social.

Organisation of the Chapters

The process of turning an interest in fun into a book has been more difficult than I had at first anticipated. Organising fun into discernible and sensible chunks—chapters—has inevitably involved compromises and omissions. Much of the book is exploratory in nature. As there has been very little in the way of systematic interrogation of fun—particularly in sociology—I intend (or hope) that this book will provide a platform for critique or enhancement in our thinking about fun, and I am not precious about assertions that are in here. I hope that people will discuss the issues raised—particularly in the spirit of advancing the capacity of having fun for others.

There are eight chapters. This introduction, a chapter on theorising fun, a chapter on fun and childhood, another on fun and adulthood, a chapter on fun at work, one on what fun feels like, a chapter on fun and recollection and a summary/conclusions chapter.

The next chapter examines fun in childhood. It starts from a historical account of the framing of fun between generations—from the Victorian era to the present day. From considering fun as a pedagogic tool to the regulation of fun in children, the complex relationship between fun as functional and fun as transgressive is discussed. Using empirical data from a variety of sources, the shifting boundaries of fun from infancy to childhood to adolescence is apparent.

Moving from the discussion of fun in childhood and adolescence, Chap. 3 discusses the ways in which fun operates in adulthood. The association with concepts of leisure is one that is often exploited in making policies to do with well-being. The chapter questions this association as meaningful to *experiences* of fun and draws explicit links with the debates on sanctioning and transgression raised in the previous chapter. Fun is presented here as being something distinct from those areas of academic interest traditionally associated with the concept—notably happiness and well-being. There is a discussion of the dichotomous relationship adults have with fun—describing it on the one hand as frivolous and ephemeral and on the other, essential to good living.

Chapter 4 discusses fun at work. There is a growing literature—largely American—on 'workplace fun'. The idea being that productivity might be increased by a concentration on creating an environment where the working day is punctuated by periods of 'fun'. This chapter starts with an overview of the efficacy of such approaches and discusses the implications for workers of the institutionalisation of fun. The chapter explores how workers experience fun and whether this bears any relation to the sorts of mechanisms employed by corporations to maximise 'workplace fun'.

The following chapter explores embodied and sensual responses as fun. It starts with a discussion about the relationship between pleasure and fun and draws distinctions between the two. After outlining debates in phenomenological and embodiment literature concerning embodied responses to the social and material environment, the chapter moves to discuss two present data from the survey conducted as part of the project on fun. These data are discussed in relation to the often-referenced 'fun' elements of activities being to do with a sensual, embodied response to them.

Chapter 6 raises the question of the points at which fun is experienced. The chapter starts with a discussion about the role of memory and recollection in reconstituting a recent past. This discussion is then used to explore the construction of fun as a post hoc phenomenon in Chap. 7. Many of the events or experiences described in studies are retold as fun. This chapter asks the question about the points at which fun is recognised.

The issue of temporality is explored alongside the idea that a narrative provides templates for understanding experiences as one thing or another but often after the event itself.

The concluding chapter brings together the key themes highlighted in the previous chapters. The distinctiveness of fun—from well-being or happiness—is reiterated, and there is a detailed discussion on the role of temporality in constituting fun as fleeting and frivolous. This is then set alongside the idea that fun is essential for a fulfilling life. This dichotomy is at the heart of the book and it is this apparent contradiction—it is argued—that has left fun outside of the consideration of sociology. There is a discussion of the relativistic nature of studying fun. The book finishes with thoughts on the transgressive in fun as being a universal principle—and that variations in understandings of fun across cultures are really variations in ideas of transgression.

A Sociology of Fun

Many of the core themes in this book are the staples of sociology. The role of culture and social interaction, our relationship to thinking, doing and experiencing and what to do with rules are all issues that have been interrogated by sociologists throughout the decades. In this regard the book is not breaking any new ground—however, the application of these areas of interest to fun is. It is unusual to find a substantive topic that is relatively untouched by academia. To realise that something as important as fun had been overlooked was exciting, and being given the time and resources to think about it has been a privilege, but also a daunting experience. When I set out to write the book, I had assumed that I would find much more literature on fun than I subsequently have. Having said that there has been a deliberate attempt to lean less heavily on literature and more on data from a survey conducted as part of this project and also on conversations that I have had with people over the past three or four years about fun and how they understand it. When Palgrave, the publisher of this book, sent the initial proposal out to reviewers, most came back with useful, but minor suggestions for shifts in focus here and there. One, however, whilst not aggressively critical, was much more strident for their suggestion as to how a book of this nature would be useful or interesting. This reviewer was much less interested in how fun could be understood or incorporated into existing thoughts about happiness on the one hand and power on the other, but wanted to know on what things people find fun, how they have it and what it means to them. It was in this spirit that the book has been written—and I hope that it is in this spirit that it will be read.

References

Becker, H. (1963) Outsiders New York: Free Press.
Bengoechea, E., Strean, W., & Williams, D. (2004). Understanding and promoting fun in youth sport: Coaches' perspectives'. *Physical Education and Sport Pedagogy, 9*(2), 197–214.
Billig, M. (2005). *Laughter and ridicule: Towards a social critique of humour.* London: Sage.
Blythe, M., & Hassenzahl, M. (2004). The semantics of fun: Differentiating enjoyable experiences. In M. Blythe, K. Overbeeke, A. Monk, & P. Wright (Eds.), *Funology: From usability to enjoyment.* London: Kluwer.
Bok, D. (2010). *The politics of happiness: What government can learn from the new research on wellbeing.* Princeton: Princeton University Press.
Brülde, B. (2015). Well-being, happiness and sustainability. In J. Søraker, J.-W. Van der Rijt, J. de Boer, P.-H. Wong, & P. Brey (Eds.), *Well-being in contemporary society.* New York: Springer.
Butsch, R. (1990). Introduction: Leisure and hegemony in America. In R. Butsch (Ed.), For fun and profit: The transformation of leisure into consumption. Philadelphia: Temple University Press.
Cameron, P. (1972). Stereotypes about generational fun and happiness vs. self appraised fun and happiness. *The Gerontologist, 12*(2 part 1), 120–123.
Canadian Index of Wellbeing. (2015). Canadian Index of Wellbeing. https://uwaterloo.ca/canadian-index-wellbeing/. Accessed 01 Nov 2015.
Churchill, S., Plano Clark, V., Prochaska-Cue, K., & Cresswell, J. (2007). How rural low-income families have fun: A grounded study. *Journal of Leisure Research, 39*(2), 271–294.
Diener, E., & Biswas-Diener, R. (2008). *Happiness: Unlocking the mysteries of psychological wealth.* Oxford: Blackwell.

Directgov. (2010). Happiness in the UK, and how to measure it. Available at http://www.direct.gov.uk/en/Nl1/Newsroom/DG_192744. Accessed 15 Aug 2011.

Fine, G. A. (1989). Mobilizing fun: Provisioning resources in leisure worlds. *Sociology of Sport Journal, 6*(4), 319–334.

Goffman, E. (1961). *Encounters*. Harmondsworth: Penguin.

Graham, C. (2012). *The pursuit of happiness: An economy of well-being*. Washington: Brookings Focus.

Jackson, S. (2000). Joy, fun, and flow state in sport. In Y. Hann (Ed.), *Emotions in sport*. Champaign: Human Kinetics.

Kelty, S., Gilles-Cortes, B., & Zubrick, S. (2008). Physical activity and young people: The impact of the built environment in encouraging play, fun and being active. In N. Beaulieu (Ed.), *Physical activity and children: New research*. New York: Nova Science Publishers.

Keppens, G., & Spruyt, B. (2015). Short term fun or long term gain: A mixed methods empirical investigation into perceptions of truancy among non-truants in Flanders. *Educational Studies, 41*(3), 326–340.

MacPhail, A., Gorely, T., Kirk, D., & Kinchin, G. (2008). Exploring the meaning of fun in physical education the sport education. *Research Quarterly for Exercise and Sport, 79*(3), 344–356.

OECD. (2015). OECD Better life index. http://www.oecdbetterlifeindex.org/#/11111111111. Accessed 31 Oct 2015.

Office for National Statistics. (2011). Measuring national wellbeing—guidance and method. http://www.ons.gov.uk/ons/guide-method/user-guidance/well-being/about-the-programme/index.html. Accessed on 30 Oct 2015.

Office for National Statistics. (2015). Measuring what matters. http://www.ons.gov.uk/ons/guide-method/user-guidance/well-being/index.html. Accessed on 30 Oct 2015.

Oxford English Dictionary Online. (2011). http://www.oed.com.ezproxy.sussex.ac.uk/view/Entry/75467?rskey=T9KbqO&result=1#eid. Accessed 19 July 2011.

Podilchak, W. (1991). Distinctions between fun, leisure and enjoyment. *Leisure Studies, 10*(2), 133–148.

Redmon, D. (2003). Playful deviance as an urban leisure activity: Secret selves, self validation, and entertaining performances. *Deviant Behaviour, 27*.

Riemer, J. (1981). Deviance as fun. *Adolescence, 16*(61), 39–43.

Rodriguez, P., Kessene, S., & Humphreys, B. (2011). *The economics of sport, health and happiness*. Cheltenham: Edward Elgar.

Roy, D. (1959). "Banana time": Job satisfaction and informal interaction. *Human Organization, 18*, 158–168.

Scanlan, T., & Simons, J. (1992). The construct of sport enjoyment. In G. Roberts (Ed.), *Motivation in sport and exercise*. Champaign: Human Kinetics.

Scanlan, T.K., Carpenter, P.J., Schmidt, G.W., Simons, J.P., & Keeler, B. (1993). An introduction to the sport commitment model. *Journal of Sport & Exercise Psychology, 15*, 1–15.

Seefeldt, V., Ewing, M., & Walk, S. (1993). *An overview of youth sports programs in the US*. Washington, DC: Carnegie Council on Adolescent Development.

Siegenthalter, K., & Gonzalez, G. (1997). Youth sports as serious leisure: A critique. *Journal of Sport and Social Issues, 21*(3), 298–314.

Stratton, A. (2010). Happiness index to gauge Britain's national mood. *The Guardian*. http://www.guardian.co.uk/lifeandstyle/2010/nov/14/happiness-index-britain-national-mood. Accessed 15 Aug 2011.

Strean, W., & Holt, N. (2000). Coaches', athletes', and parents' perceptions of fun in youth sports: Assumptions about learning and implications for practice. *Avante, 6*(3), 83–98.

Sumnall, H., Bellis, M., Hughes, K., Calafat, A., Juan, M., & Mendes, F. (2010). A choice between fun and health? Relationships between nightlife substance use, happiness, and mental well-being. *Journal of Substance Use, 15*(2), 89–104.

The State of the USA. (2015). The state of the USA. http://www.stateoftheusa.org. Accessed 01 Nov 2015.

Thomas, A. (2007). *Youth online: Identity and literacy in the digital age*. New York: Peter Lang.

Veenhoven, R. (1991). Questions on happiness: Classical topics, modern answers blind spots. In F. Stack, M. Argyle, & N. Schwarz (Eds.), *Subjective wellbeing: An interdisciplinary approach*. Oxford: Pergamon.

Veenhoven, R. (2009). World Database of Happiness: Tool for dealing with the 'data deluge'. *Psychological Topics, 18*, 229–246.

Waite, L., Luo, Y., & Lewin, A. (2009). Marital happiness and marital stability: Consequences for psychological wellbeing. *Social Science Research, 38*(1), 201–212.

Walker, C., & Fincham, B. (2011). *Work and the mental health crisis in Britain*. Oxford: Wiley Blackwell.

Wolfenstein, M. (1951). The emergence of fun morality. *Journal of Social Issues, 7*(4), 15–25.

Yee, N. (2006). The labor of fun: How video games blur the boundaries of work and play. *Games and Culture, 1*(1), 68–71.

Young, K. (2013). Managing online identity and diverse social networks on Facebook. *Webology, 10*(2), 1–18.

2

Theorising Fun

There has been very little attempt in sociology to theorise fun. There have been few concerted efforts in any discipline to theorise fun. This is perhaps because it feels antithetical to having fun to imagine that it is something that needs to be or can be theorised. We tend to have quite a naturalistic view of it as something that just happens—particularly as a result or by-product of something we think of as more tangible or susceptible to theorising, like happiness or well-being. However, it is important to situate fun theoretically, as it is with any social action or situation, in order to be able to distinguish it from other assumed positive or affective phenomena. This is a first attempt in sociology to do such a thing, but there have been notable attempts elsewhere—in psychology with Mary Wolfenstein, in leisure studies with Walter Podilchak and in Human Computer Interaction (HCI) Studies with Mark Blythe and Marc Hassenzahl in particular. With regard to this book there is a discussion of the affective or emotional utility of fun in social settings. This provides the grounds for exploring people's everyday experiences of fun. In this respect a distinct way of examining fun as related to—but not entirely dictated by—institutional relationships is suggested.

Theorising Fun: Chasing Shadows

In the course of the writing of this book I have asked many people 'what is fun?' It was one of the questions on the survey that I conducted for the study. When put on the spot very few people are able to comfortably discern precisely what it is that they are describing and how it is distinct from other things that are often associated with fun—happiness, pleasure, joy, amongst many other things. However, we use the word all the time, and seem to have an uncomplicated relationship to the phenomena that are covered by it. The aim of this chapter is to offer a template or model for how we might understand fun as a social entity in itself. This is very much the start of a conversation about what it entails and how we might best recognise, enjoy and preserve the experience of having fun. I understand that the process of theorising often feels quite reductionist, particularly when thinking about human behaviour and emotions. My intention is not to produce the definitive model, and when I present one later in the chapter, it will be clear that there is plenty of ambiguity built into it. The aim is to build on the suggestions of Blythe and Hassenzahl in suggesting that we *can* identify fun when we have it—and can say something distinct about it. However, this lack of commitment to definitive absolutes is not a weakness in my view, but a strength. A key attribute of sociology is the capacity of the discipline to accept or expose ambiguity, document apparent contradictions that inhabit the same spaces and be open about the messiness of social life.

In terms of understanding fun, it has been seen as the by-product of other emotional or social practices or experiences. In general, literature that does mention fun will do so in the context of discussing topics like happiness (Cameron 1972; Jackson 2000; Sumnall et al. 2010) or deviance (Riemer 1981; Redmon 2003; Keppens and Spruyt 2015), for example. As was suggested in the introduction, researchers have referred to fun but generally they have referred to it in relation to other things, and most commonly conflate it with enjoyment or happiness, or they have spoken about it discretely but have failed to provide an explanation as to what it is. There is a 'taken for grantedness' about fun with the expectation being that we all know what each other are talking about. Despite this, there have been attempts to think about fun and the consequences of having it. Early thoughts from Martha Wolfenstein and Donald Roy will be examined here, as will the work of Walter Podilchak from a leisure studies perspective. I will then spend some time thinking through the consequences of the thoughts of Blythe and Hassenzahl before presenting ideas that draw on many of these sources to develop further a sociological stance on fun.

Wolfenstein and Roy

The etymology of fun outlined in the introduction indicates the changing meaning of the word. Given that fun, as we might understand it, is a relatively recent semantic phenomenon, the sorts of sources that are useful to scholars of fun are fairly modern. As Martha Wolfenstein suggests, a modern sensibility to fun probably developed in the years immediately following the Second World War. This is not to say that modern fun is not heavily influenced by pre-war fun—in the UK this is particularly true of the role of social class in formulating a view of savoury and unsavoury pursuits—but with the development of leisure, increasingly expendable incomes and the marketisation of 'youth' culture, fun becomes socially more important than before 1945.

I would suggest that there have been discourses of fun that have led us to a particularly confused view of what fun is, when it is good and when it is bad and whether we need to encourage or control the fun of others. These discourses relate to the ways in which happiness and pleasure, alongside fun, have been thought about from a variety of disciplines or perspectives. From Victorian psychology and early anthropology we have a sense of the role of deviance in pleasure taking—this is then accentuated in criminological and sociological accounts of deviance and rule breaking as pleasurable. We also see the development, in leisure, of the importance of identity, power and inequalities in the ways in which we promote our own happiness and also take pleasure. In terms of isolating fun in these discourses it is really in the 1950s that a few scholars begin to think more systematically about what happiness and then fun consist of (Wolfenstein 1951; Goldings 1954; Fellows 1956).

The post-war era is important when thinking about fun because of the seismic shift in attitudes to life in general. The trauma of the war provoked a re-evaluation of the worth of life. I think that the idea that having fun was necessarily a distraction from more weighty or serious matters was weakened to the point where it was important across the social classes to demonstrate how much fun you were having. According to Wolfenstein this development rapidly brought different pressures than the pre-war requirement to demonstrate restraint or stoicism:

> Here fun from having been suspect if not taboo, has tended to become obligatory. Instead of feeling guilty for having too much fun, one is inclined to feel ashamed if one does not have enough. Boundaries formally maintained between work and play break down. Amusements infiltrate into the sphere of work, while in play self estimates of achievement become prominent. (Wolfenstein 1951: 16)

Despite having been written well over half a century ago, this excerpt brought to my mind social media, such as Facebook or Instagram, where users edit largely pictorial representations of their lives or identities in such a way as to present a face to the world that is desirous to it. A lot of energy is poured into representing fun, as opposed to just enjoying it. It is a common complaint that life is increasingly lived through a lens and many of us are guilty of doing this to ourselves. For example, social media profiles tend to overaccentuate fun as if it is constant and consistent (Strachan 2015). People tend to post, represent and manage happy occasions and exciting or wild times on holiday, at the weekend, at parties, at home, and so on. It is very difficult to represent the mundane in these media and representing life accurately is not the point. I think that, similar to the scenario described by Wolfenstein in 1951, we have developed media to demonstrate how much fun we are and how much fun we are having.

At around the same time that Wolfenstein was identifying representations of fun and the associated responsibilities—particularly for mothers—scholars of work and employment were noticing the role of distraction in industrial relations. Rather than fun being viewed as an add-on, or as a frivolous waste of time, people like Walker, Guest and

Roy were hinting at the importance of fun as both a survival strategy and a bonding mechanism between shop floor workers. In his famous paper *Banana Time*, Roy describes the necessity of overcoming what he terms 'the beast of monotony'. For him it was 'the talking, fun, and fooling which provided the solution to the elemental problem of 'psychological survival' (Roy 1959: 158). In these two areas we can see the tensions that have accompanied ideas of fun throughout the last couple of hundred years. It is essential to a fulfilling life, it is frivolous and time wasting, it is a commodity to be produced and consumed, it is important for psychological well-being, it is something to be displayed and declared however little of it we are actually having.

These sources from the 1950s are valuable, they indicate attitudes and values, however, there is no concerted effort to understand what fun is and how we know when we are having it.

Podilchak

Even though there is a comprehensive literature on play and enjoyment in psychology, the problem remains that it is difficult to know what authors are talking about with regard to fun—particularly as terms are used interchangeably or taken for granted. In leisure studies, however, there was an attempt to theorise fun in relation to enjoyment; this work was largely undertaken by Walter Podilchak in the 1980s and early 1990s. He contends that there needs to be a concentration on enjoyment and fun as being components of leisure if we are to tease out the distinctions between them. As was discussed in the previous chapter, what is most useful in Podilchak is his identification of power in fun. He says this 'fun has been undertheorised because of its explicit challenge to inequalities in social hierarchical forms and societies' (Podilchak 1991: 134). For Podilchak the levelling out of inequalities is a core component of fun—as opposed to enjoyment or pleasure which maintain social hierarchies. Similar to Wolfenstein, Podilchak notes that 'conceptions of leisure relegate to fun all socially or morally "inferior" forms of free-time interactions—whether it be drinking, informal get-togethers, "doing nothing" and fooling around, or sexual activity' (134). So the starting point for theorising fun has to be that it is considered an inferior phenomenon to enjoyment, happiness or pleasure—although related. That it has something to do with power and hierarchies—or an absence of either. That it has something to do with experiences in time—rather than something more esoteric or ethereal and that it is marked by a lack of formality.

Definitions of Fun

As I have said elsewhere, when I was first developing ideas for what became this project, I was struck by the lack of literature specifically on fun. This point was made by Walter Podilchak in 1991 also saying that when he started researching fun he was surprised at how little there was written about it—particularly in the social sciences. Despite Podilchak's observation, only a limited amount of academic writing has been dedicated to understanding fun. In this section I give a brief overview of ideas about fun before explaining in a fair amount of detail the thoughts of Blythe and Hassenzahl—Blythe edited a book with others on *Funology* [their word, not mine], which I have found particularly useful.

There are brief descriptions of fun in a variety of sources, but as with pretty much all academic references to fun, it is thoroughly underdeveloped. Wolfenstein simply describes it as 'gratification, deep, intense and isolated' (Wolfenstein 1951: 23). I like this description as it encapsulates the subjective experience of something meaningful but boundaried, temporally and embodied. In 1962 De Grazia suggested that 'fun and freedom often seem almost synonymous: when you are having fun you're free and only if you're free can you have fun' (De Grazia 1962: 423), it is distinctive in that fun is considered amoral or apolitical, whilst much free time is morally and socially contained. De Grazia advances Wolfenstein's very personal, internal explanation and highlights the social situatedness of fun. Once again the apparent contradiction of fun with phenomena within which it is placed—free time—is interesting. Despite the possibilities afforded by combining these definitions from the 1950s and 1960s, they were never properly exploited. As Podilchak suggests, in 1991, fun is undertheorised. By the 1980s any imaginative enquiry into fun had all but vanished. Podilchak reports Kelly as simply saying that fun is the 'experience of immediate pleasure' created by 'doing something'. As with other accounts, Kelly does not dwell on what fun is, but describes the conditions under which fun can occur. For them fun is interactional, and in the example of play, phenomenological, 'the person has freedom and choice to create a new potential affective identity, but it is clear that this is only an intention. The social conditions necessary for this intentionality to materialize are identified as fun' (Podilchak 1991: 135). Within this account it is the relational aspect of social conditions that are important for understanding when fun occurs. Fun is not something that can be identified in isolation to the recognition of the correct social conditions. As Podilchak notes, in Kelly's account 'fun is clearly established as a type of social relationship construction than a specific activity' (Podilchak 1991: 135). There is clearly something in this; if conditions are not correct, fun will not happen, but it is interesting to me that when questioned people do think that fun is something more tangible than just social conditions and relationships. In the subsequent chapters data will be presented that will suggest that we have quite clear parameters of not just how we have fun but what things we do are fun. That said fun does contextualise bonds between people. Those that have fun together create conditions for particular types of relationship. We are used to categorising friendships by the types of things that happen within them. Sometimes friendships, where having fun is the primary experience within them, are portrayed as less important than those where talking personally or deeply—those that have a more confessional tendency—is a prominent characteristic of the friendship. Despite the contextualisation of the bonds between people, the emphasis on the self in narratives of enjoyment undermines the role of the social and this then takes attention away from fun—a socio-contextual experience. This emphasis on the self and enjoyment relegates fun to a trivial factor in the more important pleasure/enjoyment project of the self. For Podilchak fun is a 'conscious restructuring of the social setting and its acceptance by interacting persons which produces an emotional reward, not strictly the intention to be playful' (Podilchak 1991: 136)—and this is not focussed on the project of the self.

Of course this is not to suggest that fun, enjoyment and pleasure are unrelated, and both fun and enjoyment are understood as processes of other-/self-oriented interactions, but for some of us they are distinct. Podilchak, for example, suggests that in both fun and enjoyment emotions are a common facet, but fun is a qualitative elaboration of enjoyment—fun is external, in contrast to the inner orientation of enjoyment. It is this external manifestation that accentuates the relational and contextual nature of fun. Podilchak again:

> When interactants are having fun, they are 'outside' themselves, but interactively connected with the other [sic] who are present. The feelings of fun only emerge in this social bond and require an equality condition among members. (Podilchak 1991: 145)

Fun persists, and even spreads, as long as 'interactants have deconstructed their biographical and social inequalities' and 'fun only lasts as long as these inequalities and power differentials are negated… one feels the other's presence of the situation' (Podilchak 1991: 145). Fun is deemed less serious only because the equality mechanism in human-ness challenges the ideological justification of the differentiated social order. Ultimately, in this theoretical frame, the seriousness of enjoyment appropriates fun.

The account from Podilchak is helpful, particularly in that it highlights the social nature of fun. I think we often imagine that fun is deeply personal and difficult to universalise, largely because it appears that people tend to find fun in different things. However, Podilchak is clear that it is not in the universalising of experiences but the universalising of the mechanism that we can best understand fun. It is not that we all find similar things fun, but that the way in which we can access fun—in whatever form that takes—is similar. For Podilchak it involves the equalising of power differentials and hierarchies between people, and that fun is an interactional phenomenon—involving other people. I think that Podilchak provides a useful backdrop, but I would contend that the subjective plays a more prominent role than Podilchak affords, in that the flattening of hierarchies is not necessary for fun to be had. We are more playful with power relations than is often acknowledged. There is something in vicarious experiences as fun that may be predicated on power differentials, but this will be explored later in the book.

Blythe and Hassenzahl

One group of people that did spend time trying to understand what fun is were computer programmers, and particularly computer games manufacturers. The economic imperative to understand what made games attractive to players drove interest in fun. If they could determine what fun was they could build the core components of it into their games systematically. However, as is explored in a collection of pieces edited by Blythe et al. (2004) it is not simply a case of producing fun and bottling it. In fact it is debatable whether in-game experiences are often that fun at all. Certainly observing children playing computer games I'm never really sure that they are having fun; amidst intense concentration, frustration, anxiety, adrenalin and anger, the process of game playing looks intense and focussed on objectives, but rarely much fun. Whilst it might be that my subjective experience of fun might simply look different than my children's, the consequences of any time blasting aliens or racing sports cars around city streets suggests something different. Perhaps games developers realised fairly early on that fun wasn't enough and that excitement and stimulation of any sort would be enough to shift units. This perhaps explains the relatively brief period of focussed attention on what fun is. As is often the case, there is a settling back into naturalistic approaches to fun—where the overriding sentiment is 'we don't know what it is, but we know how to have it.'

In one particular chapter in the edited collection *Funology* (Blythe et al. 2004), Blythe and Hassenzahl start to tease out the distinctions between 'enjoyable experiences' (Blythe and Hassenzahl 2004: 91), with a concentration on fun. In an attempt to synthesise what fun means today Blythe and Hassenzahl (2004) provide a rare template for theorising fun. They attempt to make clear distinctions in the relationship between enjoyment, pleasure and fun and start by pointing out the context dependency of enjoyment:

> Think of activities associated with enjoyment: sex, dancing, riding, swimming, taking drugs, playing a game, talking, joking, flirting, writing, listening to music, looking at a painting, reading, watching a play, movie, or other entertainment,. Each of these activities is enjoyable, or not,

depending on the situation that the activity is embedded in. Each situation is a unique constellation of a person's current goals, previous knowledge and experiences, the behaviour domain, and applicable social norms. A ride on a roller coaster can be enjoyable, but maybe not after an enormous dinner. (Blythe and Hassenzahl 2004: 94)

The context dependency of experiencing enjoyment exposes the subjective and emotive elements of it, and alongside pleasure, the individualised phenomenal experience becomes important to its interpretation. Fun, however, occupies a less ethereal realm than either enjoyment or pleasure to the point where fun 'has quite specific and differential everyday meanings' (Blythe and Hassenzahl 2004: 95). So for Blythe and Hassenzahl the overlaps between these three phenomena are not enough to obscure distinctions between them. For them the difference between fun and enjoyment appears to be narrower than between fun and pleasure. A key difference between fun and enjoyment is in interpreting the 'relationship between ongoing activities and states of mind' (Blythe and Hassenzahl 2004: 94). Whilst many things might be interpreted as enjoyable they might not be described as fun. The distinction between fun and pleasure is one of distraction and absorption.

Distraction and Absorption

Whilst many things might be interpreted as enjoyable, they might not be described as fun. The distinction between fun and pleasure is one of distraction and absorption. Blythe and Hassenzahl provide a model to explain this—including the obvious caveat that they are not presenting a polar dichotomy and that experiences are fluid. In this model, 'Experiential and cultural connotations of fun and pleasure' (Blythe and Hassenzahl 2004: 95), Blythe and Hassenzahl set up four dichotomies at either end of four continua. At one end are features of fun and distraction and at the other features of pleasure and absorption. They then work through each of the four continua with 'fun/distraction' characterised by 'triviality' and 'pleasure/absorption' characterised by 'relevance', next for fun 'repetition' being counterpoised with 'progression' as a feature of pleasure, 'spectacle' on a continua with 'aesthetics' and 'transgression' with 'commitment'.

They explain an essential difference between pleasure and fun, and I think to a large extent enjoyment also:

> During the fleeting and amorphous experience of fun, we are distracted from the self. Our self-definition, our concerns, our problems are no longer the focus. We distract ourselves from the constant clamour of the internal dialogue. This is not meant to imply that fun is unimportant or by any means 'bad'. Its ability to distract with short-livedness and superficiality satisfies an important psychological need. (Blythe and Hassenzahl 2004: 95)

This teasing out of differences leads then to a series of observations based around continuum between dichotomous extremes.

Triviality and Relevance

Blythe and Hassenzahl suggest that fun is 'the antonym of serious' (ibid 97) and is often an adjunct to make serious pursuits—science and art, for example—more appealing particularly to young people through distraction from the seriousness of the endeavours. In order for something to be fun there needs to be an absence of seriousness and in this sense activities described as fun are trivial. Activities that are 'absorbing' are more likely to be personally meaningful and, according to Blythe and Hassenzahl, relevant. As absorbing activities and objects assume significance for us they become 'relevant'. Relevance is derived through opportunities for personal growth, memory—meanings attached to activities, experiences or objects and anticipation—'fantasies about activities that are about to happen are a source of pleasure. In all three of these domains fun is marginalised in the attribution of meaningfulness—or absorption—to activities or objects. By outlining what fun isn't in this case, Blythe and Hassenzahl reveal what fun is—distracting, not serious and not intended to reveal anything about the self.

Spectacle and Aesthetics

According to Blythe and Hassenzahl the senses need to be stimulated by what they call spectacle. As opposed to pleasure 'attention is "grabbed"' (99). They accentuate the gaudiness, colour and wildness of fun, whilst in the aesthetics of pleasure order and abstraction are important. They say that the difference between pleasure and fun is this: 'The fun of the spectacle is a result of the *intensity* of perceptual stimulation, whereas aesthetic value is concerned with the *quality* of perception' (99).

Repetition and Progression

Another distinction between fun and other types of pleasurable experiences is that of repetition and progression. For Blythe and Hassenzahl the idea of progression is inherent in forms of pleasure but not in forms of fun. They suggest that as popular culture is 'concerned with cycles of sameness, endless variation within self-replication', so is fun. There is no particular movement forward or challenge in fun as there is in other forms of pleasure—the fun in games, for example, is in the joy of a repeated act.

Transgression and Commitment

This distinction is perhaps the most widely understood or acknowledged. The idea of transgression, in the form of rule breaking, is often cited as fun in of itself. Once again Blythe and Hassenzahl illustrate an idea of fun by outlining its corollary. So for them 'transgression can be fun but commitment may be pleasurable' (99). Being absorbed or committed to an activity involves acceptance of assumptions and rules surrounding that activity—in the example they choose, two players of a game experience it differently depending on their orientation to the rules. One gains pleasure by adhering to the rules and enjoys playing properly. The other gets bored and tries to cheat to make the game fun. Both enjoy themselves but in different ways—one through commitment and the other through transgression.

Blythe and Hassenzahl are clear that the relationship between fun and other positive affective states are not discrete—there are crossovers between happiness, pleasure, fun and enjoyment—and these crossovers make distinguishing between these phenomena difficult. Also, it is clear that in developing the model they are not setting up stark dichotomies and that experiences travel along a scale between, for example, transgression and commitment. It is perhaps this lack of distinction, allied with the marginalisation of the discourse of fun, that has obscured it as a subject worthy of sustained consideration.

Schema of Fun

In the summer of 2013 I developed a final year undergraduate module at the University of Sussex called 'A Sociology of Fun'. In this module 20 students and I spent three hours a week over a four-month period trying to figure out what fun is, and how we experience it. We read much of the literature that is represented in this book, shared stories, interviewed others and talked and talked and talked. I will say that it was the most rewarding teaching experience that I have had. The students entered into the spirit of the project with open minds and a sense of adventure in their scholarship. I was clear with them from the outset that as there was very little written about fun, and almost nothing sociological on fun. As a result, one of the objectives of the course was to start to write a sociology of fun. Our initial discussions revolved around how best to theorise fun. As is explained above, we used Blythe and Hassenzahl's thoughts in a chapter in the edited collection *Funology* (Blythe et al. 2004) as our starting point—and it has remained an important touchstone throughout this project.

Through discussion and debate, often using Blythe and Hassenzahl's 'Experiential and cultural connotations of fun and pleasure', we developed what we think is a more nuanced account of how fun might be theorised and then put in to some sort of schema. As with all tables it is irredeemably reductionist, and I am sure that some people will find gaps in any account that uses it to make definitive statements about the nature of any experience—is it fun or not? However, there is a deliberate ambiguity in the descriptions of each element and I hope that criticism of it will seek to enhance, clarify or refute in order to develop a more full account of what fun consists of and how we can recognise it.

Unlike in the Blythe and Hassenzahl case, the schema presented here does not describe extremes along continua. Moreover, it describes relationships between elements that are supportive of each other—or will simply point out that the combination of elements results in experiences or sensations that can be described as fun. Another thing to stress is that I am not suggesting that there is anything absolute in the ways that we experience fun. If we do something that does not conform to every element of the model suggested here, then that does not mean that we are not having fun—some things may be present and others not, but as an agglomeration of the discussions that 21 of us had over a number of months—informed by previous thoughts on fun, happiness and pleasure—this was the result (Fig. 2.1).

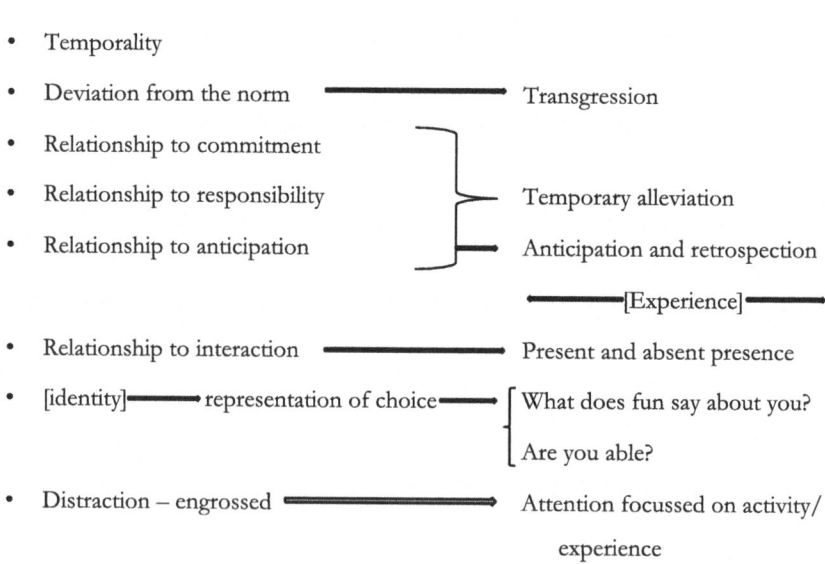

Fig. 2.1 Schema of fun

Temporality

This is an element missing from Blythe and Hassenzahl as an explicit item. Fun experiences sit in time in a way often distinct from happiness or pleasure. It tends to be the case that fun starts and stops and we can identify quite accurately in time when this is. It does not resonate or echo in time in the way that happiness and, to lesser extent, pleasure can. This precise location in time is important for the future identification of what might be fun. When whatever it is starts, the fun starts; when whatever it is stops, the fun stops. When describing fun, children often conflate it with play, and this is an important step on the road to precisely locating fun as something that starts abruptly and stops abruptly, in ways that happiness or pleasure do not.

Deviation from the Norm and Transgression

Deviation from the norm generally equates to something out of the ordinary. This may include Blythe and Hassenzahl's 'exciting goings on' (2004: 92), but also incorporates things that are not associated with the normal train of events or experiences. Fun tends to disrupt routines, even if it establishes its own routines (see Roy's *Banana Time*). Crucially this deviation from the norm can provoke transgression of some sort. This is similar to Becker's definition of deviance, where it is simply 'the infraction of some agreed upon rule' (Becker 1963: 8). Transgression need not be some sort of grand statement; it may simply mean not really doing what you are supposed to or what you normally do. When it comes to work fun will be away from productive tasks, when it comes to time at home it will be away from domestic chores and when it comes to normalcy it will be periods of abnormalcy.

Relationship to Commitment: Temporary Alleviation

Commitment here is defined in the way used by Blythe and Hassenzahl. It involves 'being absorbed or committed to an activity' and 'involves acceptance of assumptions and rules surrounding that activity'.

Unlike Blythe and Hassenzahl I tend not to think of commitment as on a continuum with transgression at the other end, rather an orientation to task or experience that is then temporarily suspended during the times at which we have fun.

Relationship to Responsibility: Temporary Alleviation

As will be illustrated later, an important aspect of fun identified by people when questioned about it is escape from present concerns or anxieties. During fun attention is directed away from responsibility towards a more carefree attitude—however short-lived that may be. It is not necessarily the case that fun is defined through irresponsibility but that responsibility is not a concern during periods of fun.

Relationship to Anticipation: Anticipation and Retrospection in Experiences

Anticipation operates in multiple ways in fun. In the moment, anticipation of what will or ought to happen next is suspended—assumptions about how 'normal' a situation is are not present. However, at the same time there is often an assumption that a situation that has been experienced as fun will be fun once more. We can recognise a situation, or even a sensation, and then anticipate that it will be fun not because of a prediction of what will happen but because of an identification with something that has *already* happened—a fun experience in the past. In this way, retrospection works with anticipation to create an openness to a situation as fun.

Relationship to Interaction: Present and Absent Presence

Generally fun is had with other people. For most of us part of fun is sharing or communicating the positivity of an experience with an other or others. Whilst many people will suggest that it is possible to have fun by yourself, it is often with reference to an absent presence—something that a person used to do/has done with someone else, or that they enjoy communicating to others after the event. Having fun by oneself is further complicated by the routine conflation of terms and concepts between fun, happiness, pleasure and contentment. However, it is not the case that people experience fun as an entirely solipsistic experience.

Identity: Representation and Choice

Identity is an important component of how we experience fun and what we think is fun. As will be explored later, fun is not just something that is a phenomenal experience. It has social resonance. The sorts of things a person finds fun says something about them. Fun is gendered, classed, culturally mediated, manifest in national identities, subculturally expressed, subjectively experienced amongst many, many other things. As such what we find fun but crucially what we profess to find fun has resonance for identity—the game of darts has a particular profile in British national consciousness, to suggest that this is something that is fun carries with it connotations, what sorts of other things you might enjoy, the company you keep and other things that you might find fun. Darts can be great fun to play as a child in a bedroom, as an adult it can be fun to play if you are comfortable in pubs, for example—you may play for something different to do in the pub or you may be a serious player. If you are a serious player, the extent to which the activity is fun is dependent on the context. Losing a high-pressure league game when you have not been playing well is not much fun. For increasing numbers of middle-class people darts is a source of ironic or transgressive fun—'people like us don't normally enjoy this sort of thing'; for large numbers of people that have grown up in families where the pub is important and darts has been played the implications of fun on identity are different. The choices that are made in the declarations of what is fun for a person demonstrate to others what sort of a person you are and in turn permit judgements and behaviours towards others on the basis of what is professed to be fun. For many a person saying how much fun it was to be involved in football violence will tell you all you think you need to know about them.

Distraction: Attention Focussed on Activity/Experience

In the distraction away from everyday or normal experiences we become absorbed in the distracted activity or experience. As we become engrossed we stop concentrating on peripheral concerns—it is this process that explains first the idea people have of being immersed in activities and second the difficulty we have to articulate what fun feels like when we are having it. Whilst we are experiencing fun we are engrossed in it to the point that it is almost impossible to then accurately reflect what it feels like. If you start thinking about fun whilst you're having it, you start doing something else—thinking about fun rather than having fun. As will be discussed in the chapter on phenomenal fun there are occasions where this might not be the case—the example of a shared experience of euphoria when dancing with someone has been mentioned as a time where the moment of having fun is recognised and explicable and the recognition is part of the fun.

Conclusion

As has been mentioned, theory is important to framing understanding social phenomena. It is through theory that things can be judged or interpreted alongside each other, and similarities and distinctions become clear. By using Wolfenstein, Podilchak and Blythe and Hassenzahl in particular a model of fun has been developed that attempts to represent the various factors that are present in fun. A criticism that I anticipate is that it is too loose on the one hand, and too restrictive on the other. How can something that talks about relationships but does not define the paths of those relationships or the intensity of them say anything pertinent about the phenomenon that the model is supposed to represent? As I have suggested, inherent in all social action and experiences is ambiguity. Ambiguity that speaks to Weber's catch-all fix of 'ideal types' (Weber [1904] 1971: 63–7) and also the ambiguity inherent in generalising an individual's experiences or perspectives. On the other hand, I anticipate some to suggest that the model is too restrictive, too many experiences of fun fall outside of the parameters of the model or lots of fun fulfils only elements of it. To this I reiterate the observation that all models that seek to describe the social are reductionist and should be open to critique; however, the schema of fun is not suggesting that you can make totalising statements about fun. It is about recognising relationships that may help distinguish fun from other social phenomena.

Wolfenstein, Podilchak and Blythe and Hassenzahl all demonstrate the importance of theoretically addressing fun. In Wolfenstein we are exposed to issues of morality and obligation—two things not often associated with fun. I do not know whether she was a feminist or read de Beauvoir but her concentration on gender and subsequent interpretation of how fun becomes subverted into obligation for mothers highlights the role of the social in constructing how we are supposed to have and provide fun. In Podilchak we find an attempt to account for the role of power and hierarchies. His ideas about the equitable distribution of power and the flattening out of hierarchies in moments of fun talk to an overtly structural account of this subjective experience. Blythe and Hassenzahl provide a systematic interpretation of how we experience fun, and also a template to start building more complex inferences about how we have fun in contrast to experience pleasure, enjoyment or happiness. These are important theoretical observations that further our capacity to understand fun. It is worth noting also that the contextual nature of the phenomenon highlights the social aspects—in particular sociality and interaction; temporality; transgression; temporary alleviation form commitment, responsibility and anticipation; identity and distraction—the identification of which is the result of theoretically informed reflection.

Over the course of the next four chapters data from the fun project will be presented, and these data should be understood in relation to the characteristics described above. In this a view of fun as being prey to all sorts of associated—and not necessarily positive—aspects of social life becomes apparent.

References

Becker, H. (1963) Outsiders New York: Free Press.

Blythe, M., & Hassenzahl, M. (2004). The semantics of fun: Differentiating enjoyable experiences. In M. Blythe, K. Overbeeke, A. Monk, & P. Wright (Eds.), *Funology: From usability to enjoyment*. London: Kluwer.

Blythe, M., Overbeeke, K., Monk, A., & Wright, P. (Eds.). (2004). *Funology: From usability to enjoyment*. London: Kluwer.

Cameron, P. (1972). Stereotypes about generational fun and happiness vs. self appraised fun and happiness. *The Gerontologist, 12*(2 part 1), 120–123.

De Grazia, S. (1962). *Time, work and leisure*. New York: The Twentieth Century Fund.

Fellows, E. (1956). A study of factors related to a feeling of happiness. *The Journal of Educational Research, 50*(3), 231–234.

Goldings, H. (1954). On the avowal and projection of happiness. *Journal of Personality, 23*(1), 30–47.

Jackson, S. (2000). Joy, fun, and flow state in sport. In Y. Hann (Ed.), *Emotions in sport*. Champaign: Human Kinetics.

Keppens, G., & Spruyt, B. (2015). Short term fun or long term gain: A mixed methods empirical investigation into perceptions of truancy among non-truants in Flanders. *Educational Studies, 41*(3), 326–340.

Podilchak, W. (1991). Distinctions between fun, leisure and enjoyment. *Leisure Studies, 10*(2), 133–148.

Redmon, D. (2003). Playful deviance as an urban leisure activity: Secret selves, self validation, and entertaining performances. *Deviant Behaviour, 27*.

Riemer, J. (1981). Deviance as fun. *Adolescence, 16*(61), 39–43.

Roy, D. (1959). "Banana time": Job satisfaction and informal interaction. *Human Organization, 18*, 158–168.

Strachan, M. (2015). *A study of happiness and the self on Instagram: Representations and the impacts on consumers*. Unpublished undergraduate thesis. Sociology dissertation module. University of Sussex.

Sumnall, H., Bellis, M., Hughes, K., Calafat, A., Juan, M., & Mendes, F. (2010). A choice between fun and health? Relationships between nightlife substance use, happiness, and mental well-being. *Journal of Substance Use, 15*(2), 89–104.

Weber, M. ([1904] 1971). The ideal type. In Thompson, K. & Tunstall, J. (1971) *Sociological perspectives*. Harmondsworth: Pelican.

Wolfenstein, M. (1951). The emergence of fun morality. *Journal of Social Issues, 7*(4), 15–25.

3

Fun and Games: Childhood

Fun is often touted as an important component of modern childhood. It is represented as an inalienable right for children to have fun. The degree of fun we are supposed to have in childhood distinguishes this phase of life from all others. The range of ways in which fun is understood in childhood is wide and frequently contradictory. At one extreme we find the widely held belief that fun is an important pedagogic tool—through having fun and playing children tend to consolidate learning more effectively—at the other extreme fun is represented as something disruptive and in need of control. It is often the case that fun is regulated by spaces—some are appropriate to have fun in, others not, by time—there is a right time and a wrong time to have fun, or it is regulated by other people. Children have to learn the rules of fun if they are to have it without interference from adults. This process of training is never more apparent than in schooling. Since the 1960s the teaching of very young children has been underpinned by fun and discovery as core pedagogic principles. When the brain is at its most gymnastic and able—in early childhood—we acknowledge that fun is an extremely effective way of fixing learning and encouraging 'learning by doing'. Associated with this is play, and, as will be explored later, play and fun are often synonymous in the minds of children in ways that are distinct from that in adults. However, as we progress through school the fun becomes marginalised and compartmentalised, as does the play. The fun has to make way for the serious stuff—but the serious stuff is actually not the content of learning but the *style* of learning. There are many ways to learn the same thing. As they progress through school years, children are coerced into understanding fun as something that does not occupy much of the day and that sober concentration is much more important. Whilst some may consider this an overly pessimistic picture of schooling, nobody that I have spoken to during the course of my thinking about fun has argued that their experiences were radically different. This is not to suggest that we are necessarily unhappy as a result of this sequestering of fun—just that it is interesting that it happens. Famously Ivan Illich (1971) suggested that this is another example of society imposing the values of traditional productive labour, control and deference upon generation after generation of youngsters, all being trained to behave themselves so as not to disrupt the power and privilege that dominates society. This process is not, of course, designed and maintained by identifiable and conscious individuals; rather, it becomes the way in which we do things—in much the way described by Norbert Elias in 'The Civilizing Process' (1939). As we get older the places and spaces in which we are allowed to have fun become fewer. We get hung up on the age appropriateness of fun and regulate our behaviour accordingly. A young woman I spoke to told me a story about how, when she was 13, she went on a trampoline and was having great fun until she noticed that some other children of about the same age were laughing at her. It transpired that they were giggling because bouncing on trampolines was something that younger children did. She never went on a trampoline again.

The confused relationship that we have with fun as we get older is clear in the ways in which we can understand it as worthwhile and to be encouraged in the example of early schooling and an unwelcome distraction and something to be controlled in the example of later schooling. The institutionalised response to our having fun is functional or transgressive. What is interesting about this, however, is that these are not actually rationales for having fun for people having fun—they can be the consequences of having fun, or fun may be the result of them, but they are rarely the impetus. Even in the example of transgression, the motivation for having fun may well be excitement or an adrenaline rush—the fact that these things can be experienced by breaking certain rules is neither here nor there, it is the sensation that is being sought—it just so happens that smashing windows and running away, for example, can stimulate these sensations.

When thinking about fun and childhood, considerations of play dominate academic writing. Although not directly addressing fun, the question 'what is play for?' is a pertinent one when trying to discern how children experience fun. The presumed association between play and fun is important to the continued struggle adults have with trying to organise and regulate children's fun. As I have suggested, an obvious example is 'fun learning' in schools. The less oppressive rote learning and more learning through enjoyment and experience that has developed over the last four decades is to be welcomed but there is still a doubt in my mind that the relationship between play and fun is as automatic as we assume. Fun and play are distinct in the same way that pleasure, happiness and fun are related but distinct. When it comes to pedagogy, there have always been efforts made to establish learning objectives—things that adults think are important for children to achieve—as something that children will want to engage with. As Martha Wolfenstein illustrated in 1951:

> Recently a ten-year-old boy showed me one of his school books. It had the title 'Range Riders' and showed on the cover a cowboy on a galloping horse. The subtitle was 'Adventures in Numbers'; it was an arithmetic book. The problems involved cowboys, horses, and so on. The traditional image of the American schoolboy has been that he sits with a large text book propped up in front of him, a book representing the hard tedious lesson which he wants to evade. And inside the text book he conceals a book of wild west stories, detective stories, or the like, which he is avidly reading. These two books have now been fused into one. I do not know whether this succeeds in making the arithmetic more interesting. But I have a suspicion that it makes the cowboys less exciting. (Wolfenstein 1951: 23–4)

This quid pro quo described by Wolfenstein is provoked by a belief that play and fun can be *for* something—in this case, learning. As will be illustrated a little later, there is often a tension between play as fun—and implicitly an end in and of itself—and play as instrumental to other development.

This chapter will address some issues surrounding play, but will also draw on the data gathered during the course of this project—where participants were asked to recollect instances of fun in their childhood—and if they are children to recall recent instances of fun. In keeping with the remainder of the book the data will be important for detailing the ways in which fun is manifest in people's lives. The experiences that are highlighted here tell us much about not just how we have fun but also how discourses of fun and social expectations play a role in mediating our experiences.

To start, however, it is worth noting debates and discourses that have developed regarding childhood as an important life stage—free of responsibilities, carefree and a time to be cherished.

The Development of Childhood

More than anybody the French historian Phillipes Aries highlighted the question of the cultural context of childhood. He points out that childhood is neither a historically nor a geographically stable phenomenon. For Aries the separation between youth and adult, as we understand it, did not exist until the seventeenth century at the earliest when changes in economic and social conditions in Europe provoked a gradual development of the idea of childhood as a distinct phase of life in a way that we might recognise (Aries 1962). He suggests:

> It is as if, to every period of history, there corresponded a privileged age and a particular division of human life: 'youth' is the privileged age of the seventeenth century, childhood of the nineteenth, adolescence of the twentieth. (Aries 1962: 29)

For Aries the medieval conception of the child was as a small adult. As soon as the child was not reliant for survival on its mother it passed into a phase of life synonymous with productivity and adulthood. However, from the seventeenth century, in France, the concept of child separates between the child within families, where parents begin to distinguish children's behaviour as a source of vicarious pleasure and amusement, and the child outside the family where, as Cunningham explains, 'moralists ... stressed how children were fragile creatures of God who needed to be safeguarded and reformed' (Cunningham 2005: 6). Aries identified education as a primary force in changing attitudes to childhood. Driven by a moralist agenda the idea of schooling being for children made clear the distinction between them and adults. As schooling spread, and the age at which a person stayed at school increased, so did the length at which a person was considered a child—so today childhood extends as far as schooling, and this is much further than it did in the seventeenth century. However, alongside the development of the idea of the specificity of schooling for children came the other puritan obsession—reform and punishment. Whilst the narrative of childhood as being a time where within the concept of family children were to be cherished, outside of the family children became creatures in need of 'order and discipline' (Cunningham 2005: 6). This translated for generations of children into physical abuse in the shape of beatings. So, for Aries it is not just the experience of being a child that is mediated by structures that are not simply observations of biology, but the *facts* of childhood that are also prone to interpretation and reinterpretation from generation to generation. There have been many critiques of Aries since the publication of *Centuries of Childhood* (1962), some accentuating methodological frailties in his analysis (Forsyth 1976; Steinberg 1983) and others disputing the emphasis Aries places on certain aspects of medieval social life (de Mause 1974; Shorter 1976). Most controversially, Aries claim that 'in medieval society the idea of childhood did not exist' (Aries 1962: 125) has come under sustained attack (Pollock 1983; Wrightson 1982). Amongst historians and social scientists concerned with childhood Aries' assertions have caused great discussion—to what extent did the industrial revolution transform child–adult relations? What is the role of social class in determining attitudes and behaviours towards children? How has parental love manifested in child–adult relations over the years? However, generally the malleability of stages of life to context is not really in dispute. The extent to which the socio-historical context influences views of childhood is in debate, the idea that it has an influence is not. Despite this acceptance that childhood changes with age and context there is still a strong biological determinism in how children are understood. To a certain degree the place where biological and social observations on childhood meet is in a close relative of fun—play.

Play

There is an inherent ambiguity in play that has interested and perplexed scholars from many disciplines:

> 'The most irritating feature of play' says Robert Fagen, leading animal lay theorist, 'is not the perceptual incoherence, as such, but rather that play taunts us with its inaccessibility. We feel that something is behind it all, but we do not know, or have forgotten how to see it'. (Sutton-Smith 1997: 2)

For Fagen the mystery of play is something that we may leave behind. His idea that we may have forgotten how to see play appeals to the sense that it is a mystery revealed to children and we lose sight of it as we grow older.

In 1962 Jean Piaget published *Play, Dreams and Imitation* (Piaget 1962) and alongside Leo Vygotsky provides complex accounts of the experience and utility of play in childhood. In a similar way to fun, Piaget suggests that play is an orientation towards a behaviour, rather than a behaviour itself or set of activities:

> Play is, in reality one of the aspects of any activity... the prevalence of play among children is therefore to be explained not by specific causes peculiar to the realm of play, but the fact that the characteristics of all behaviours and all thought are less in equilibrium in the early stage of mental development than in the adult stage, which is, of course, obvious. (Piaget 1962: 147)

He then goes on to contest certain assumed preconditions of play and sets out conditions that are met when a person is playing. The first, and most useful for the purposes of considering fun, is that play is an end in itself. This is a key distinction between play and work, where work does not contain the end in the activity. There are four further conditions: play is spontaneous whereas work involves compulsion; play is an activity for pleasure whereas work is not; play involves a lack of organisation whereas work is highly organised and structured; finally, Piaget suggests that play involves freedom from conflicts—where children involved in play transcend the conflicts of everyday life and imagine scenarios where material constraints or anxieties are no longer present. He concludes:

> It is clear that all the criteria suggested in order to define play in relationship to non-ludic [spontaneous or playful] activity result, not in making a clear distinction between the two, but rather stressing the fact that the tonality of an activity is ludic in proportion as it has a certain orientation. (Piaget 1962: 150)

It is interesting that Piaget persists in characterising play as specific to particular activities and interactions. This is despite having suggested that play is an orientation to activities. As will be illustrated, this confusion also occurs when thinking about fun.

Attempts by psychologists in the 1950s and 1960s to explain play have dominated discussion of it ever since, but as is often the way, the early pioneers of research could not account for inconsistencies in their theoretical frames. Smith and Cowie point out that there always appear to be caveats when trying to tie down play:

> Play is often described as an 'active' behaviour (yet not all play is physically active) it is described as characteristic of infancy and childhood (yet adults play, even if it is often with children); and as behaviour which is easily suppressed by other motivations, such as hunger, fear or anxiety, curiosity, or fatigue.... This has led to a functional definition of play, that the behaviour has no immediate benefits or goal. (Smith and Cowie 1991: 170)

The role of utility in thinking play is important, particularly when considering the problem of lack of specificity inherent in attempts to define it. A recurring theme in psychological and educational writing about play is that it does serve a practical *developmental* function. This developmental function does not sit comfortably with one of Piaget's conditions of play: that it is an end in itself. If play is an end in itself it is difficult to understand what elements of this self-contained phenomenon are useful for development. There is often talk of the development of motor skills or hand–eye coordination but these skills are acquired in a variety of settings and contexts. Smith and Cowie characterise play as having a lack of focus but the persistence of evolutionary perspectives in studies of play steers us towards more functional, biological explanations for how and why we play. Susan Isaacs suggests that play is essential to both cognitive and emotional growth and her evolutionary view leads her to observe that animals that learn more play more. Whilst many of the biological and evolutionary explanations may offer some level of understanding the pertinence of Piaget's conditions of play suggest more interesting social questions. There is a balancing act highlighted by Wolfenstein—where the developmental function of play as identified by adults has to appeal to the unreflexive, unselfconscious play of children. As I will illustrate with the data gathered for this project this is the same as with fun.

The issue of development has interested scholars of play from the outset. The contradiction implicit in the self-defining characteristic of play running alongside developmental functioning exercised Vygotsky and Piaget.

The relationship between play and learning was vociferously demonstrated by Vygotsky who suggested that play is 'the leading source of development in the pre-school years' (Vygotsky 1966: 6). Reminiscent of Piaget, Vygotsky suggested that the nature of pretend play is to liberate children from the immediate constraints of a situation into a 'world of ideas'. So, according to Vygotsky, play has a dual role in the early lives of people—it is necessary for the acquisition of skills and provides a space for liberation from the material concerns of 'real' life. But this does not leave much space for any idea of fun or frivolity. I suppose levity could be found in the imaginative world that, according to Piaget, transcends the world of everyday conflicts but there is no account in these writings of what fun does in play.

In *The Ambiguity of Play* Sutton-Smith talks about fun as being considered the 'essence' of play for many scholars of childhood and play (Sutton-Smith 1997: 187). It is fun that draws together disparate approaches to play. He suggests that despite their differences many writers on fun seem to understand fun as an explanation of 'why players want to play' (Sutton-Smith 1997: 188). In 1983 Rubin, Fein and Vandenberg carried out what would now be called a systematic review of literature addressing issues of play. They then summarised how they understood the intersections between various approaches and authors. Broadly there were six key features of work on play that spanned most of the material examined. This work was undertaken in 1983, and Sutton-Smith provides a critical commentary about each of these points in *The Ambiguity of Play* (1997) but in the course of researching this book I have found that all six are still strongly representative of how scholars understand play. This is not to suggest that they are correct or incorrect, simply to note that they have become firmly embedded as principles for understanding play.

1. The first is that 'the hallmark of play is that it is intrinsically motivated', in other words, play is fun. As might be anticipated by the dominance in the field by Vygotsky and Piaget, there appeared to Sutton-Smith a preponderance of psychologists espousing this view. He points out that many anthropologists and historians would have a problem with this intrinsic motivation to play given that there is a view that much play was extrinsically motivated 'by village requirements' (Sutton-Smith 1997: 188)
2. In accord with Piaget, there is a strong contention that 'play is characterised by attention to means rather than ends'. Sutton-Smith suggests that this is related to a Cartesian characterisation of the dualism of work/play. However, he suggests that play involves 'multiple personal and social goals as well as solely instrumental play behaviours' (Sutton-Smith 1997: 188). Once again, play is doing some work. When it comes to fun I can't help thinking this insistence on instrumental worth is such a strong habit that it becomes almost impossible to imagine anything in life that does not possess it—I am not convinced.
3. The next category is that 'play is guided by organism-dominated questions'. For Sutton-Smith, once again, this assertion involves a misinterpretation of discrete elements of social life. As with his disquiet about play operating in a goal-free vacuum, he points out that we can play when we don't appear to be—sitting at a desk our minds might be at play whilst the task being materially performed is not play. For children all sorts of things are play. So 'the realities of play involve a more complex mixture of organismic and contextual behavior [sic]' (Sutton-Smith 1997: 189)

4. A strong discourse in play literature is that play is supposed to be non-productive and non-instrumental. For Sutton-Smith this ignores the complexity of everyday 'intentionalities' (Sutton-Smith 1997: 189). For him this is another attempt to involve a dualism between work and play that is not as clear as we think. It is interesting to note that either way this contention is viewed, it places fun in an odd position. For many people, fun and the associated good feelings are an instrumental by-product of play. So, if Rubin et al.'s position is accepted, then play does have an instrumental thrust but if Sutton-Smith's position is accepted, then the instrumentality of play might still be quite distinct from our views or experiences of work.
5. The fifth element of play research identified by Rubin et al. is that play involves 'freedom from externally imposed rules'. Sutton-Smith simply points out that much game playing is dependent on rules and that a lot of play is oriented around rules that have been applied by other players or pre-exist the play, as in established games. It is interesting to think of this point in relation to Blythe and Hassenzahl's observation about transgression and commitment when it comes to fun. One person is getting pleasure from playing the game properly and their opponent is having fun secretly cheating.
6. The final feature is that 'players are actively engaged in their activity'. For Sutton-Smith this ignores vicarious play or daydreaming as play.

For Sutton-Smith the concentration of fun as a distinct arena of experience has been overstated. He consistently points out the interconnectedness of experiences and feelings—he is uncomfortable dealing in the psychological certainties often iterated in writing on play. Of particular interest to this study is the idea of fun as an essence of play, and whilst a counterpoint is suggested by Sutton-Smith it is from anthropological and historical perspectives that are not themselves interested in the experience of fun as much as what it does socially. In this respect the relationship between intrinsic motivation to have fun and the interconnectedness of experiences and feelings becomes fraught. Many of the observations made by Rubin et al. in 1983 persist in the ways we think about play, and consequently fun, today.

Play and Fun in Empirical Studies

As is suggested above, play and fun are both characterised as involving a lack of objective, and both are thought of as being apart from serious pursuits. Generally, they are also understood to be related but not necessarily dependent on each other. It is possible to play without having fun—I think that this is particularly true in adulthood and sport. There is no doubt that a game of squash is play but my experience is that it is rarely fun. It seems that in order to make sense of play we give it some sort of productive value—particularly in childhood. It is imbued with developmental, cognitive, ecological, biological and social worth and without play many of the developmental stages through which we pass are not fully realised.

This does beg the question what is it for in adulthood—but this will be addressed in the next chapter.

In order to make sense of fun we tend to give it an instrumental, developmental purpose. It has to be *for* something, and whilst this might be partially true it could be equally the case that it can serve as a useful distraction from activities that are *for* something. A theme that will be picked up later, particularly in the chapter on work, is that fun is deployed to deflect us from serious and productive concerns. I think this is an adult projection onto the lives of children. An instrumental view of play—or fun—sounds like a set of theoretical explanations made to conform to a mature, adult world view—one that is not possessed by children. I'm not sure it matters what play or fun is for, what matters is that it is experienced and enjoyed by children. There are relatively few studies where children have been asked directly what fun is or how they understand their own experiences of fun, but there are examples where researchers have attempted to test theories of fun on children in designing computer interfaces (Read et al. 2002; Sim et al. 2006) and adults have been asked how they imagine children experience fun in engagement with sports (O'Reilly et al. 2001). None of these examples give any sense of how children feel about fun.

An interesting discussion on what children counted as 'play' was carried out in Canada by Glenn, Knight, Holt and Spence. In this research they found that almost all activities could be defined as play—a great example provided by one child:

> I like to play with cats and dogs. I like to play on my Wii. I play soccer in my backyard.... I like horses. I like to ride my bike and I like to build snowmen. (Glenn et al. 2012: 6)

Rather than play being a discrete or focussed activity it appeared as though the context within which activities took place was important to an activity or circumstance being identified as play. There was also corroboration of Vygotsky's observation that in play the means were more important than the end—play is self-contained. However, the most striking aspect of the research was this observation about how the children saw the relationship between play and fun:

> Through their discussions, the children articulated what it was that led to certain activities being playful. The overriding consensus was that play was fun. As soon as an activity was not fun it was no longer considered play. (Glenn et al. 2012: 190)

The mutual inclusivity that the children in this study afford the concepts of fun and play once again provokes the question of why fun has been so roundly ignored as an important area of study, particularly in childhood studies. I wonder whether the developmental and biological explanations for why we play do not sit comfortably with the frivolousness and pointlessness often viewed as defining characteristics of fun. However, it would appear that fun has an important place for children in maintaining participation in play. Glenn et al. go on to acknowledge that children have a different agenda when talking about play, but there is no attempt to explain what the children understand fun to be—the very thing that distinguishes play from non-play in the study.

The lack of care in using fun as a mechanism for saying something about play is common in academic writing about play and young people. Broner and Torone, in their examination of playfulness in language (Broner and Torone 2001), claim that fun is an experience of positive affect that is often associated with laughter. Something done for fun is something that is not meant to be taken seriously—in other words something that is not real, genuine or sincere. (Broner and Torone 2001: 364)

This is a fairly ropey definition, but they then go on to say that fun is a component of language play and rhymes, puns, nonsense are important in the pedagogy of language and concept development (Broner and Tarone 2001: 364–5). There are many studies accentuating the importance of making sport and physical recreation fun for children and young people (Bengoechea et al. 2004; Jackson 2000; MacPhail et al. 2008; Scanlan and Simons 1992; Seefeldt et al. 1993; Siegenthalter and Gonzalez 1997) and none of them provide any useful explanation as to what is meant by fun and how it is to be understood either by the research participants or by the readers of these pieces of academic writing. The underdevelopment of theories of fun has been highlighted earlier, and will be a consistent theme throughout this book, but it is not helpful to give such scant attention to a concept that is then going to be a component of grand claims—but this is what seems to happen to fun routinely.

Data from the Survey

As has been mentioned, a major part of this project was to try and get people to tell me what they thought about fun. Much of the work about happiness, and what there is about fun, tends to be theoretical. With a couple of exceptions (e.g., Kerbs and Jolley 2007; Glenn et al. 2012) there is not much of a sense in the literature of how people more generally understand or define these concepts. Much of the rest of this book will be given over to the results of a survey conducted in the spring and summer of 2014 where 201 people answered open questions about their experiences of fun in childhood; those that were adults were asked about adulthood and also what fun felt like and also how fun was different from happiness or pleasure. The reason for the survey, and the reason that much of this book will document the results, is that fun is had by people, and as a way of reorienting theory—to make sure that it is doing what it should—it is important to ask people how they experience the world and what they think about it.

Respondents to the Fun Survey were asked to 'Tell me about an occasion in your childhood where you had fun (if you are still a younger person tell me about a time when you were even smaller)'. Almost all of the stories fitted with one of the following: adventure, family, friends, holidays, the outdoors (nature, open space, water), play, make-believe and building. Despite this relative uniformity, the responses to this question were wonderful in their description and invocation of happy memories for people—and I will present quite lengthy quotes from some of them because of their richness. This sentiment shone through most of the contributions and on the surface each appears unique to the person—they have to be, it was their experience, nobody else's. However, on closer inspection patterns began to emerge in the subject matter and the combination of features of the stories that were being left with me.

Adventure

When recalling instances of fun in childhood many people told stories or made statements that related to a sense of adventure—this was directly:

> I think about how me and my brother would ride our bikes around town, in the country, and things would just happen. Like getting caught on the railway bridge and having to hang below the rails while the train passed over or launching our corrugated iron boat and me being saved by my brother when I was sucked into quicksand. Adventure might sum it up. (F71. Retired school teacher)

And indirectly:

> When I was about 12 or 13, I went on a camping holiday in the Lake District with my family. A large part of the holiday was games or activities organised by the holiday company. One evening, the holiday-goers (adults and children) were driven on a minibus to a lake with a small island in the middle. A member of staff then told us that on the island there were guerrillas (I, of course, heard 'gorillas') guarding a captain who

needed to be freed. The aim was to be dropped on to the shore, split up, find the captain and return to shore with them. We then boarded a little boat and were taken to the island. We then played what was basically an island-based game of cops and robbers. If the guerrillas caught us, we were taken to the prison and had to wait to be rescued. It got slower darker, and after an hour or so one side or the other won, and were ferried, and then driven, back to camp. It was probably the most exciting game I ever played. And it was really, really fun. (M22, Student)

In different ways both of these accounts invoke a sense of adventure. In the first the infusion of transgression and danger accentuates that adventurous spirit whereas in the second the 'out of the ordinary' scenario and location adds to the excitement and adventure. Generally, the responses that I thought captured adventure fell into three categories. Stories that involved dusk or darkness, stories of naughtiness and stories where grown-ups were absent.

Adventure: The Dark

There were a number of accounts that took place in the dusk or in darkness. Children are not used to being up late and so playing or doing something as it gets dark in places that they normally only see in daylight—or being awake when they are normally asleep—adds something to the specialness of particular times and also to the transgressive nature of the experience. In answer to the question about occasions of fun in childhood a woman that works in a supermarket said:

> When we used to go camping. We used to do a lot of haven holidays, sometimes in a caravan, sometimes in a tent, but we have been to Tenby in Wales, Weymouth and West Bay were favourites though [sic]. We used to play card games and board games, which would be really fun because Mum and Dad used to play with us too. We used to use torches and tell each other scary stories. We used to go on late night forest walks, or beach walks. (F21, Shop worker)

As I have said many of the quotes have covered many themes; however, the adventure implied in late night forest or beach walks is what

I want to highlight here, and also the explicit role of parents in making this happen. Holidays feature large in many of the accounts and as such parents and siblings are often integral to these memories and experiences. However, friends or peers are also present:

> When I was ten I went to a sleepover at a friend's house (a birthday party, I think). We stayed awake until around 2 a.m. and ate a 'midnight feast' at midnight. The whole event was fun because going to bed with my friends there was such a novelty (this had always been a solitary activity previously), and being allowed to stay up late felt like a real privilege. As someone who has a very sweet tooth (this has continued into adulthood!), eating chocolate and sweets at midnight felt like the biggest treat ever, especially with all my friends there. (F31, Lecturer)

It is worth noting at this point the role of others in the fun being reported in this part of the study. Almost all of the stories involved other people—only 4 of 201 respondents told stories where they were by themselves and had fun. As I have said, I am not suggesting that more people do not have fun by themselves, but when asked to isolate an experience of fun in childhood almost everybody mentioned other people.

With reference to darkness others spoke about playing later than usual, 'playing in rivers and being let out until it got dark' (M49, Decorator) and 'playing football all afternoon with my best friend and into dusk in the rain and diving around' (M43, Social Worker).

The dark represented the 'out of the usual' for many people. It provided a context for Blythe and Hassenzahl's 'exciting goings on' (Blythe and Hassenzahl 2004: 92). There is a deep association in our imagination about the dark or the night-time as mysterious and perhaps unpredictable. For children this is an intoxicating mix, so when we are allowed as children to spend time in the dark—particularly out of doors—it touches many of the elements that we associate with fun.

Adventure: Naughtiness

As with the first quote from the retired school teacher, many of the stories involved elements of naughtiness or transgression/rule breaking, and in that people were expressing fun. Again, in common with the first quote a couple of people mentioned railway lines as particularly fun places to play. Another theme in naughtiness was groups of children. An example being a researcher in Scotland who explained 'me and my friends used to go to 'explorations' in the countryside close to where we lived. We'd pack up lunch and go out for the day, climbing over fences, getting muddy, running away from cows' (F29, Researcher). Another person said, 'I remember having a lot of fun as a child. It was mainly outside—we had a lot of children in the neighbourhood so we ran around, rode bikes and stole apples from neighbouring gardens. Lots of things were fun' (F39, Academic). Both of these examples imply groups of kids kicking about an area going where they wanted—stealing apples (or scrumping where I grew up) and having to escape cows suggest that they were having fun in spaces that they were not supposed to be.

Adventure: No Grown-Ups!

I am always interested to hear adults explain how much better their experiences as children were when there were no adults around—particularly as we increasingly insist that our children are supervised or kept indoors under the gaze of adults. I think that this is sad—and there are plenty of people that are attempting to reverse this inexorable slide into increased surveillance and control (see, e.g., Gray 2013; Brussoni et al. 2015). Bearing this in mind there were several people that highlighted an absence of adults in their accounts of fun. From parties when parents were away to wandering about in the summer holidays—freedom from adults underscored accounts of fun, a nice example of a synthesis of several themes where an absence of adults was key as given by a person that worked in a bar in Brighton when she said:

> The things I remember having the most fun doing were more adventurous activities such as climbing trees, cycling, especially being alone in the countryside with friends, without parents being around. (F24, Bar staff)

Adventure, outdoors, friends and no grown-ups create the conditions for fun in the memory of this person. Another example of this sort of synthesis was provided by researcher when he said 'We went on holiday to North Wales and [my] sister and me met another brother and sister who we played with for a week. I remember this was fun because there were no parents around and it was fairly unusual for us to meet other kids on holiday' (M37, Researcher). In this extract the importance of other children and being on holiday is accentuated by the absence of adults.

Family

It was initially a surprise to me how many people mentioned family when recounting stories of fun in childhood. I had anticipated that friends would dominate the narratives, but on reflection, given the importance of home and holidays to children, it should not have been such a surprise. Grandparents and parents were obviously important, but so were siblings. I like this as it challenges the stereotypical narrative of warring brothers and sisters. These contributions are wonderful to read, often underwritten with love and affection.

> When I think of the fun I had as a child I think mostly of days out and holidays that we had as a family. My grandparents would almost always come with us and we had lots of laughs together. In particular I remember a fortnight spent at Pontins Pakefield. It was 1976, the weather was hot and sunny and my brother, sister and I were allowed the freedom to go off and do the things we wanted without being tied to our parents—the Bluecoats would look after us—but the family would do stuff together too—playing cards, swimming, donkey derby, dancing, organised team games. (F45, Research Officer)

Holidays and family came up again and again:

> When we used to go to on beach holidays in the summer, my parents would advise my brother and I to 'try and dig a hole to Australia' in the sand. This was very clever of them—it would keep us occupied for much of the day, and was always great fun! I think we genuinely thought we might make it all the way down to Australia, with our little colourful plastic spades. (F33, PhD Student)
>
> My Grandparents would take us to Hastings seafront every summer along with my cousins, Aunties/Uncles. We'd have a meal all together, usually fish

and chips, they'd all give us all 2ps and 1ps to use on the arcade machines and I remember never wanting it to end. (F24, Sales Assistant)

Clambering over rocks at the beach where my grandparents lived, days spent with my brother. Endless competitions to be fastest, most daring or do the silliest walks, and then attempts to dam the water as the tide went out. (F37, Teacher)

One particular respondent gave a pertinent view of fun in childhood from a rare position—that of a great-grandparent:

Learning to swim in the sea, and being on my Dad's shoulders when he dived in off the pier, and told me to open my eyes and look at what was going on under the water. When my own children were young, we had fun making up plays for the puppets we made, playing hide and seek in the woods and cornfields, and shouting messages from the downs to the house, and looking at all the push button exhibits in London museums. Then I had fun all over again with the grandchildren, playing shops with anything we could find, telling them stories, and seesawing, pushing the roundabout to go faster. Some Great Grandchildren, who don't have Gameboys and Xboxes, give me so much fun, telling me jokes, and playing almost the same type of games I played with their mothers, and making me laugh with their efforts at looking after me. (F86, Retired Keep Fit Teacher, Voluntary Worker, Speaker)

Whilst it is not entirely like the other quotes—in as much as the great grandmother talks about her adult experiences with her children, grandchildren and great-grandchildren, it does offer an insight into a continuity of fun having between generations. Despite differences in the machines of play—and her clear antipathy towards Gameboys and Xboxes—children enjoy similar types of fun across generations.

Family: Parents

Parents were people to have fun with as well as facilitators of fun, and figured largely in the stories of fun in childhood. I think that it is a testament to the parents of those that responded to the survey that it is with them that, when asked, people chose to recall fun times. That might seem a bit soppy, but it was a happy surprise that so many people have positive memories of their folks associated with fun. I would anticipate that they would be present in narratives of love, happiness or security—but I hadn't assumed that they would be so prominent in stories of fun.

The inventiveness of parents in making fun was clear in many of the stories:

> In the school holidays my mum used to take my brother and I to the park—often Richmond Park and we would go exploring; at the time there were terrapins in the ponds as well as the usual deer, birds etc. We would take a picnic and find a tree, climb as high up it as we could and have our lunch in a tree—this would be called a 'tree-nic' and became a summer tradition that my mum still reminisces about now. (F26, Proofreader)

And in accord with Blythe and Hassenzahl's observation about repetition, another said:

> I used to really like going to Gatwick Airport for day trips with my parents and my cousin or a friend. We would watch planes, ride on the monorail, play airhockey, visit the Warner Bros store where they had a basic touch screen computer game and sometimes eat at a restaurant. I liked that it felt like a little holiday. The trips started after my Dad volunteered on our school trip there in year 9. (O28, Student)

In both of the last two quotes part of the fun was the repetition of something that was out of the ordinary—and it happened with parents. The parents were clearly confident that these events were fun for the children and, as was suggested in the chapter on *Theorising Fun*, anticipation, repetition, temporality, triviality and transgression all work together to produce times that are fun. There were other stories that paint a more familiar picture of fun times with parents like 'swimming with my parents in the sea when young' (M55, ICT Consultant) or 'going to the local park with my parents on a Sunday afternoon when we were little and playing "What's the time Mr Wolf?" with Dad who would chase us all over the park' (F49, Academic). There were other lovely little vignettes, 'being thrown up and down in a clean sheet, coming off the washing line, held by a parent at each end' (F42, University Professor) and 'going for a bike ride with my parents at the nearby park. I think it was my first time riding my bike without my stabiliser wheels so I felt like "Oh, I'm so grown up now!"' (F20, Student).

Over a quarter of the stories from respondents to the survey mentioned family members as the people that they remember having fun with as a child. That is not to say that they were not present in other testimonies in the survey—just that family members were mentioned explicitly.

Friends

About a quarter of respondents also mentioned friends. As I keep saying, having fun is something we do with other people and friends are clearly important throughout our lives. They play an integral role in our fun having. As fun is a social activity that we have with people that we are positively oriented towards it is no surprise that friends feature heavily in narratives of childhood.

There have been examples that I have used to illustrate other features of the data—sleepovers, playing on railways—and there were many examples of fun that involving groups of kids. As a researcher in the Midlands said 'whenever I remember my childhood and the fun aspects of it I think about time spent with friends, so I would say fun was to me spending time, playing with my friends' (F30, Researcher). Being outdoors with friends featured, and as will be mentioned later, building and creating sprang to mind for some respondents when asked to tell me about an occasion in their childhood when they had fun. However, several people mentioned being at their own or others' houses.

> Going round to a friend's house after the after-school club, our mothers would sit and chat, we'd play. I remember laughing so much cola would come out of my nose. Those Friday evenings were brilliant, 10p cans of pop and 5p bags of crisps, the ghetto blaster, 4-coloured light bulbs, dancing to Vanilla Ice. Never mind the craft/sport activities we did before. Spending the time after at my friend's house is something I'll never forget, staying up late and watching comedy on Channel 4. Brilliant. (F33, Facilities Co-ordinator)

> When I was younger 10 yrs circa, me and my friends used to set up obstacle courses in my house climaxing in the descent of the stairs using duvets, sleeping bags and other materials. It sticks out cos no matter how many times we did it, it was always immensely fun. (F21, Student)

Predictably enough play and friends also featured, with games—'playing murder in the dark at a friend's house aged around 8 (F39, Teacher); 'playing hide and seek with friends in the neighbourhood' (M24, Student), but playing in the street seems to have been important for many. An economist said that they spent time 'organising and playing mock "Olympics Games" with friends on the street that I lived as a nine-year-old. We competed against each other in a variety of fun events' (M30, Economist) and a physical therapist living in the USA said 'I had fun playing outside after school with my friends from the street. We'd play 2 man hunt or on bikes or on bikes or up at the school. I liked physical games because I was fast. I liked my 'street' friends partly because they were not in my class at school' (F38, Physical Therapist). Another person said:

> When we were about 5–12 we used to play in the wooded area opposite our house. [There was] a gap of about 20 m that ran along the length of our street. We used to play run outs and camps etc. Would spend all day there [sic] and pop home for food. There was about 9 of the kids in our street that was in the 'gang'. Very fun times. (M39, Fire Fighter)

A Research Assistant said 'being outside—building treehouses, cycling. You didn't need to go far away—simply playing outside with my friends in my street are my main memories of having fun as a child' (F26, Research Assistant).

Holidays

As is evident in the other categories, holidays were mentioned often. These periods of time are set up for discrete experiences of fun. Holidays are already out of the ordinary and rules are often relaxed during this time—the opportunity for spontaneity or excitement is exacerbated by not being at school.

Many of the quotes listed above—digging in the sand to Australia, night walks with torches, playing slot machines in Hastings—were all instances of fun had on holiday. There is a clear crossover between family and holidays as categories when it comes to fun. As children we tend to go on holiday with our families. It is gratifying to think that the time and money spent on going on holiday with children is, for the most part, well spent. There were several people that did not go into much detail but simply said things like 'collecting mushrooms on holiday' (F39, Academic), 'going on annual holidays to Wales and spending days on the beach, digging holes in the sand and swimming' (M47, Carer) or 'living in a caravan with mum and cousins in the summer' (F57, University Professor). There were others that were as pithy but a little more specific; 'when I was about 7, during a family holiday to Bournemouth, we all went to Bovington Tank Museum' (M44, University Lecturer) or 'playing rounders with my family on Orkney' (F36, Researcher).

There were occasions in the data where issues elsewhere in the respondents' childhoods were ameliorated by occasions of fun, particularly on holiday. A student from Kent said 'I went on a family holiday in 2000 (making me 2) and we went walking near Snowdonia every day together without arguing…much.' (F20, Undergraduate Student). Holidays were also opportunities for fun making on their own terms for children who tended to be a little more introverted. As a lecturer from Brighton said:

> Hard to pinpoint one occasion, but family holidays. These were in Britain when I was primary school age. Actual fun was probably going out for the day somewhere new, buying souvenirs and playing with my sister. However I also liked the chance to have quiet time to read so I think that mixture made holidays fun for me. I wasn't a confident child so occasions with lots of other children, like birthday parties were quite anxious experiences for me, rather than fun. (F36, University Lecturer)

Overall, it is noticeable that holidays are defined, for children in the UK at least as times out of school, and this is where most of the fun happens. As was suggested earlier, something happens in schooling where fun and play are considered important to learning in very early years and then filtered out of schooling to the point where, for many 16-year-olds, the classroom is the least fun place imaginable.

Outdoors

Of 201 respondents to the survey 150 mentioned being outdoors. It appears that, overwhelmingly, in narratives of childhood the outdoors is a place where fun happens. It has been mentioned to me a couple of times that I might get different responses in terms of locations of fun if I had surveyed children only. The presumption being that many would have mentioned computers or online experiences. Whilst I cannot say categorically that this would not be the case, I would contend that as fun is a social experience people of whatever age will identify times with other people—whilst this can happen online with virtual communities, but not in the same way as in the 'real' world.

Outdoors obviously incorporates a large number of subcategories or codes and I suppose an assumption might be that the coherence in the data that I claimed earlier is an artefact of my coding, but the responses broke down fairly neatly into relatively few subcategories, given the amount of responses. Also, the crossover between categories was large. Under the rubric of outdoors fell gardens, nature, open space and water. I organised nature under the headings animals, the sea and trees. The open spaces were the beach, parks, the street and woods.

Nature: Animals

Animals figured prominently in the stories of childhood fun. Several people mentioned horses. An undergraduate student said:

> The first time I got to go horse riding when I was 5. I had always wanted to go horse riding but my parents wouldn't let me until I learnt how to ride a bike. So I learnt to ride a bike and had my first lesson. I really enjoyed that experience, so much that I am still riding 16 years later. It's also an experience I vividly remember, probably because of how much fun I had. (F21, Student)

A couple of people mentioned pets; one particularly nice story was provided by another student:

When I was about 5 I remember having a lot of fun cruising around the neighbourhood in my pink corvette power wheels with my hamster in the passenger seat. I thought to myself, 'when I grow up I'm going to get a car just like this and fill it full of hamsters.' (F29, Student)

In combination with holiday a student advisor said a particular memory of fun in childhood was 'helping with the harvest on holiday on a farm ... ending the day by making a den in a barn out of hay bales—finding a cat that had kittens was an added bonus' (F49, Student Advisor at FE College).

It was interesting that there were relatively few pets mentioned. The occasions that dominated these stories tended to involve encounters with animals that accentuated the unusual circumstance that the respondents had found themselves. Most common was encounters with animals during holiday times.

Nature: The Sea

Many people talked about the experience of being in the sea. Swimming and body surfing were mentioned either as core elements of moments of fun or as the memory of fun times. These sorts of generalisations were relatively common in the data as I am sure you have noticed. An example in this section came from a textile designer who said, 'When I was 6 or 7 my mum and dad took us on a cheap holiday to Devon, and I remember having so much fun watching the sheep racing in the street and going swimming with my mum and dad' (F23, Freelance Textile Designer). Whilst there is a level of specificity in time in this sort of story, it is not an instant per se:

> Had so many occasions. I grew up in Southern California, and a day at the beach was a favorite [sic]. I loved going body surfing, chasing and catching waves. Ever since I can remember, I collected seashells, so after I had tired myself out in the sea, I would spend all evening scouring for shells. (F59, Plant Area Manager at a Garden Centre)

The ways people used the sea were often similar in the data:

> My outlet for fun during childhood was surfing, first on a boogie board and then later (starting around age 14) board surfing. This is 'serious fun'—takes a lot of focus and energy but I spent hours and hours in the water. I have many memories of that, hard to choose just one. (F35, Lecturer)

Surfing or body boarding was mentioned by several other people. As with other accounts the role of family is important to the fun being described at the beach:

> Camping/caravan holidays—going to the beach everyday with my immediate family as well as cousins and uncle. BBQs with my Dad and Uncle, fishing and crabbing. Going in the sea with my siblings and cousin on rubber rings and a blow up boat, certain occasion that was fun was when my sister and brother dragged me and my cousin out to sea and left us, was scary but very funny. (F21, University Student)

Other people said things like 'On family holiday. Lovely sunshine. Swimming in the sea in Scotland' (M50, Researcher) and 'swimming with my parents in the sea when I was young' (M55, ICT Consultant).

Nature: Trees

Trees featured in many accounts as important for having fun. It is interesting that they feature in stories as props for fun, and whilst the stories are not specifically about trees, it is striking how often they feature as a coincidental feature or a site of having fun. Some comments mentioned trees in passing, 'I had fun playing with my friends, particularly in parks or on our bikes, or climbing trees. I had fun doing art related activities or just running around being silly' (F22, Student) whilst for others trees were integral to the story. A parent talked about 'playing in the woods and making dens' (F45, Stay at Home Parent).

Open Space

Many people, about a quarter of respondents (26%), talked about having fun in what I have called 'open space'. These spaces included the beach, parks, fields and forests. The association with outdoors, space and freedom is palpable in these accounts. A university tutor said:

> Clambering over rocks at the beach where my grandparents lived, days spent with my brother. Endless competitions to be fastest, most daring or do silliest walks, and then attempts to dam the water as the tide went out. (F37, University Teaching Staff)

Another person said:

> Playing 'Fox and Hounds' with children from my street. The game would last for hours and range over local farmland and bracken fields. These games reached their zenith the year we all got walkie talkies. (M41, IT Technician)

There are many things that are unspoken, but can be assumed from most of the stories involving open space. Unless the weather is bad it is rarely mentioned and it is not unreasonable to assume that stories involving beaches or parks will also have involved fine weather. However, there were other instances of fun that did not necessarily rely on the weather. A lecturer said 'Drayton Manor Park—log flumes with my Nan' (F37, Senior Lecturer) and whilst it may likely that the weather was good enough to encourage Nan onto the log flume, it is not a necessity. Another example of the sorts of ambiguities that lead us to fill in the gaps is found in this story:

> When I was about 10 years old, I went with one of my friends and his family to a playground in Tredegar, South Wales. Unexpectedly they had an enormous rope climbing frame there which I spent several hours climbing on. I had never seen anything like it before—it amazed and exhilarated me. I talked about it for months afterwards. (M37, University Lecturer)

Another person said 'playing up a mountain on a swing with all my friends' (F20, Student). The importance of filling in the gaps is that it enables us to identify more closely to the experience being conveyed. As the swing on the mountain with friends is all I know I imagine the scene—the landscape, the length of the swing, the weather, the friends. In imagining it I bring the experience into frames of reference that chime with my own expectations for the condition of fun having. To a certain extent this is what is happening with many of the stories of fun in childhood. The relative uniformity of the accounts ensures that the fun is positively communicated to others—and the identification with a particular type of childhood and a particular type of person is maintained.

Nature: Water

Accounts from the beach clearly involve water. What was interesting, however, is that relatively few of them actually explicitly referred to water. There were plenty of other scenarios that did mention it. Amongst other mentions of rivers a student in Sussex talked about 'swinging on a rope swing over a river with my friends all day long' (F44, Student). Pools in gardens also inspired several accounts, and whilst they are not strictly products of nature, water is—so I have included it here:

> When I was little, my parents set up a 4 foot pool in the backyard for my sister and I to play in. We would swim for hours. I think the only thing I wore that summer was a swimsuit. We had the best time. (F28, Crafter/Artist)

An IT engineer in the south of England talked about being a child and having fun in Australia:

> I grew up in Australia. I remember going to the community swimming baths on hot summer evenings, when it was very hot in the day, they used to open the pools late. I t would be a nice, balmy evenings [sic] with lots of people there. I remember we used to have certain sweets that we would buy, and soft drinks, and just hanging out in the warm evening at the swimming pool with friends and family. (M54, IT Engineer)

Others were more inventive when creating pools; a student remembered:

> Making a splashing pool out of a plastic sheet and bits of plank, playing with my brother in it, shaping landscapes and creating islands in it. (Trans22, Student)

Outdoors: Gardens

Gardens featured as a place where fun was had, particularly with reference to friends that lived nearby. There were references to tree houses, slides and games but paddling pools in gardens featured prominently in stories of fun in gardens.

Another student talked about the role of imagination in their paddling pool fun:

> Playing with my best friend in her back garden. Role playing games, where we'd be lost in our own invented worlds, we got the sprinkler out (one that points up vertically) and pretended that it was a portal to another world. We used the blue plastic paddling pools like shells that everyone used to have and pretended it was a boat. (F19, Student)

Whilst a researcher and parent highlighted the role of perceived risk and transgression:

> I have a terrible memory but what comes to mind (probably prompted by photos) is dressing up and driving around the swimming pool in our trikes in our garden (we lived in the tropics) pretending to be adults, the fun came from the adrenalin rush of nearly falling into the pool and giggling about being grown ups. (F43, Part-time researcher and full-time Mum to Toddler Twins)

Play

A fair number of people (17%) identified play in their fun having in childhood, and these accounts ranged from stories of impromptu play through to organised sport. In accord with stories elsewhere in the data there were several themes highlighted in short sentences. An example was provided by a student in south-east England:

> Playing with other kids outside, laughing a lot. Coming home feeling exhausted and satisfied, smelling like outside. This in summer [sic], when the window is open and the warm air comes in. (F26, Student)

This vignette touches on the social aspect of fun, laughter, contentment, being outdoors, a visceral sense of fun, home, the weather—and crucially play. For many people play was the axel around which fun spins. As a researcher said 'whenever I remember my childhood and the fun aspects of it I think about time spent with friends, so I would say fun was to me spending time, playing with friends' (F30, Researcher), another simply said 'playing—lived in a village and roamed all over' (F39, Academic). There were mentions of the chasing game 'fox and hounds', 'hide and seek' and stories of games organised in the streets by gangs of children. Plenty of play took place on the beach and in parks—and many of these specific examples have been highlighted earlier. There were also a few references to organised play or sport (5%). As might be expected, football featured, but also gymnastics, rugby, surfing, shooting and skiing were also mentioned.

Play: Make-Believe

For a particularly childish sensibility towards fun the accounts of make-believe were striking. Fewer people than I had anticipated referred explicitly to make-believe (9%) but those that did offered a glimpse of experiences that struck a chord with me at least. There were pretend scenarios, 'pretending to be in a band' (F38, Lecturer), 'imagination games/playing out pretend scenarios—house, school, shops' (F28, Graphic Designer) to more elaborate accounts; 'when my cousins and I went to each other's houses we would make up plays/stories and spend hours practicing them before performing in front of our parents and grandparents' (F20, Student). A professor said:

> Taking all my teddies and dolls in a toy pram with my friend Jane from over the road to the park for my teddy to marry my teenage doll

(name of Rita). My mum made us dolly sandwiches to take and we probably had some cake as well, cannot say for sure but was probably about 8. (F58, Professor and Head of Department)

Whilst most of the adults that responded to the survey remembered occasions of fun between the ages of 8 and 14, there were a few that recounted much earlier memories. A couple of those were in the section on make-believe. An administrator said:

I remember having particular fun at the age of four-five at pre-school. We were playing at a tea party and I was bossing everyone around! I also had my pull along horse for show-and-tell (grew up in the States) so it felt like a special day. (F33, Administrator)

The overriding sense from these narratives, however, is of getting lost in the stories that we invent to play:

Playing 'Cowboys and Indians' up the 'Rec' [recreation ground] when the grass had been mown and left in big rows one summer and I could crawl along as an 'Indian' which I always preferred being, and 'shoot' the cowboys. Idyllic. (M69, Retired FE lecturer)

Playing with my best friend in her back garden. Role playing games, where we'd be lost in our own invented worlds, we got the sprinkler out (one that points up vertically) and pretended that it was a portal to another world. We used the blue plastic paddling pools shaped like shells that everyone used and pretended it was a boat. (F19, Student)

Building

Building emerged as a theme with 8% of respondents talking about physically constructing as fun. On the whole these were accounts of den or 'house' making—'playing in the woods with friends making dens' (F45, Stay at Home Parent); 'messing about with friends, including two imaginary friends. Making dens. Making mud baths. Telling stories. Role play. Building Barbie houses. Sport.' (F41), 'rope swings and making dens are particularly fun moments' (F47, Overworked Lecturer).

Fun and Childhood

This chapter is a bit of a mish-mash of theories that touch on related or embedded issues—the nature of childhood and play—and data largely harvested from memories of childhood. I understand that this is problematic to a comprehensive account of how children have fun. However, as Glenn et al. (2012) point out, it is difficult to discern from children where the distinctions between phenomena are. As has been mentioned, for most children in their study there was mutual inclusivity between fun and play as though they are the same thing rather than separate entities that, in childhood, map onto each other very closely. As we get older the separateness of play and fun becomes more and more obvious—you can have one without the other. It is this that occludes fun as being of distinct interest, particularly as play has been associated with developmental phases in children. If play and fun are understood as pretty much the same thing and the need for play is seen to diminish over the life course then it is little wonder that fun has escaped serious attention. It has been irrevocably associated with childhood and the lack of seriousness and responsibility that comes with such status.

However, fun plays a pivotal role in orienting ourselves to relationships and cultures of childhood that we then carry for the rest of our lives. Many of the memories here are portrayed in terms of warmth and positivity—and this is what fun does. A consistent theme throughout this book is that fun must be important, as imagining a life without fun is to imagine something bleak and dystopian.

It is strange that having acknowledged the importance of fun in childhood that we filter it out of our everyday experiences of each other as we get older. The role of fun in pedagogy feels particularly instrumental and antithetical to how most of us understand fun in childhood. As was suggested earlier, fun is recognised as important for early years' learning—at the time when our brains are at their most agile and creative. As we progress through schooling the fun is filtered out of our 'day to day' experience of education until by the time we are 16, for most of us, the classroom is about the least fun place in which we spend any time. This is not the fault of teachers but of an education system where outcomes are marked often by an absence of creativity or joy. In much the way that Illich argues that timetabling students at school is a way of creating a workforce that operates on the timeframes of others, a cynic might say the same of fun. As fun is sequestered from the school experience to smaller and smaller discrete sections of the day, we develop a sensibility towards it as had in small doses and at appropriate times—and those times are controlled by somebody else. Perhaps this explains the importance of transgression to modern fun—there is very little time for legitimised fun, so we make fun of the process of legitimisation. That said, I think that there has always been something transgressive or naughty about many forms of fun.

The themes that were identified in the data were surprisingly congruent with each other I felt. The outdoors, family, friends, holidays, adventure and play came up time and again. The locations where fun happened were also strikingly similar—parks, gardens, beaches, wooded areas. But it is also interesting what did not appear. There were hardly any mentions of what I would call organised fun—outside of sport. There were almost no theme parks or computers. There were very few accounts of fun indoors. The childhood fun iterated here was organic, messy, imaginative, transgressive, social and joyful.

The relative uniformity within the accounts reflects two things. The first, most obvious point is that the majority of the accounts derive from a particular cultural standpoint. Most of the respondents were living in the UK at the time at which they answered the questionnaire (87%) and, whilst there was a good spread of ages, the large majority of respondents were between the ages of 20 and 50 (79%). The second point is that this relatively homologous group have similar ways in understanding how fun is best communicated and best understood—this could be particularly true of the predominantly middle class profile of the respondents. It is not just fun, but also the communication of fun, that is culturally mediated. In order that others can recognise the fun being described it needs to register as fun to the listener. There are occasions where this relationship breaks down and an event or experience being explained as fun by one person is not recognised as fun by the other. In this instance there is a cost to both parties—what sort of a person finds *that* fun? / what sort of a person doesn't think that's fun? This disjuncture speaks to ideas of identity and the sorts of judgements that are inherent in Wolfenstein's 'fun morality'. This is not to disavow the experiences being communicated in the survey or to suggest that respondents did not actually experience the things they told me about as fun, but it is interesting that there was so much more uniformity in the accounts than, say, the accounts provided by the same respondents to the question 'Tell me about a recent occasion when you had fun?'. So, part of the problem here is that the accounts have been largely drawn from the memories of adults. A future project will concentrate exclusively on under-18s, and discern how children and young people are understanding the fun that they are having in situ. As with much of the lives of youngsters I suspect that many of the preconceptions about the differences between young people and 'grown ups' will not be realised and they/we are more similar that adults care to acknowledge.

References

Aries, P. (1962). *Centuries of childhood: A social history of family life*. New York: Random House.

Bengoechea, E., Strean, W., & Williams, D. (2004). Understanding and promoting fun in youth sport: Coaches' perspectives'. *Physical Education and Sport Pedagogy, 9*(2), 197–214.

Blythe, M., & Hassenzahl, M. (2004). The semantics of fun: Differentiating enjoyable experiences. In M. Blythe, K. Overbeeke, A. Monk, & P. Wright (Eds.), *Funology: From usability to enjoyment*. London: Kluwer.

Broner, M., & Tarone, E. (2001). Is it fun? Language play in a fifth-grade Spanish immersion classroom. *The Modern Language Journal, 85*(3), 363–379.

Brussoni, M., Gibbons, R., Gray, C., Ishikawa, T., Hansen Sandseter, E. B., Bienenstock, A., et al. (2015). What is the relationship between risky outdoor play and health in children? A systematic review. *International Journal of Environmental Research and Public Health, 12*(6), 6423–6454.

Cunningham, H. (2005). *Children and childhood in Western society since 1500* (2nd ed.). Harlow: Pearson Longman.

de Mause, L. (1974). The history of childhood. *History and Theory*, XII.

Forsyth, I. (1976). Children in the early medieval art: Ninth through twelfth centuries. *Journal of Psychohistory, 4*, 31–70.

Glenn, N., Knight, C., Holt, N., & Spence, J. (2012). Meanings of play among children. *Childhood, 20*(2), 185–199.
Gray, P. (2013). *Free to learn*. New York: Basic Books.
Illich, I. (1971). *Deschooling society*. Harmondsworth: Penguin.
Jackson, S. (2000). Joy, fun, and flow state in sport. In Y. Hann (Ed.), *Emotions in sport*. Champaign: Human Kinetics.
Kerbs, J., & Jolley, J. (2007). The joy of violence: What about violence is fun in middle school? *American Journal of Criminal Justice, 32*, 12–29.
MacPhail, A., Gorely, T., Kirk, D., & Kinchin, G. (2008). Exploring the meaning of fun in physical education the sport education. *Research Quarterly for Exercise and Sport, 79*(3), 344–356.
O'Reilly, E., Tompkins, J., & Gallant, M. (2001). 'They ought to enjoy physical activity you know?' Struggling with fun in physical education. *Sport Education and Society, 6*(2), 211–221.
Piaget, J. (1962). *Play, dreams and imitation*. New York: Norton.
Pollock, L. (1983). *Forgotten children: Parent—child relations from 1500 to 1900*. Cambridge: Cambridge University Press.
Read, J., MacFarlane, S., & Casey, C. (2002). Endurability, engagement and expectations: Measuring children's fun. *Interaction, Design and Children*. Available at http://chici.org/references/endurability_engagement.pdf. Accessed 03 Nov 2015.
Scanlan, T., & Simons, J. (1992). The construct of sport enjoyment. In G. Roberts (Ed.), *Motivation in sport and exercise*. Champaign: Human Kinetics.
Seefeldt, V., Ewing, M., & Walk, S. (1993). *An overview of youth sports programs in the US*. Washington, DC: Carnegie Council on Adolescent Development.
Shorter, E. (1976). *The making of the modern family*. Michigan: Basic Books.
Siegenthalter, K., & Gonzalez, G. (1997). Youth sports as serious leisure: A critique. *Journal of Sport and Social Issues, 21*(3), 298–314.
Sim, G., MacFarlane, S., & Read, J. (2006). All work and no play: Measuring fun, usability and learning in software for children. *Computers and Education, 46*(3), 235–248.
Smith, P., & Cowie, H. (1991). *Understanding children's development* (2nd ed.). Oxford: Blackwell.
Steinberg, L. (1983). *The sexuality of Christ in Renaissance art and in modern oblivion*. Chicago: University of Chicago Press.
Sutton-Smith, B. (1997). *The ambiguity of play*. Cambridge: Harvard University Press.

Vygotsky, L. (1966). Play and its role in the mental development of the child. *Voprosy Psikhologii, 12*(6), 62–76.

Wolfenstein, M. (1951). The emergence of fun morality. *Journal of Social Issues, 7*(4), 15–25.

Wrightson, K. (1982). *English society 1580–1680*. London: Routledge.

4

Fun and Frivolity: Adulthood

Moving from the discussion of fun in childhood this chapter discusses the ways in which fun is understood and experienced in adulthood—but also addresses issues of transition from adolescence to adulthood in relation to fun. It is clear that most people think that we experience fun differently in adulthood than we do in childhood—things that were once boring become fun: sunbathing, shopping, chatting, drinking, relaxing in a spa, gardening, reading the paper on Sunday, watching the Antiques Roadshow, for example[1]—fun as adults, not much fun as children.. It is an accepted wisdom that we grow into some forms of fun and grow out of others. That said, there is a strong discourse that some forms of fun in adulthood can be a return to a more innocent or childish sensibility—or that in fun we can escape from the responsibilities or burdens of adulthood. The multidimensional and context dependency of fun again complicates attempts to say something definitive about it. However, it is the context dependency of it that may give us clues to how the idea of fun is constructed differently in adulthood—even if this difference between fun in childhood and fun in adulthood is not experienced so distinctly.

---

[1] I am aware that this is not a definitive list.

For my own part I clearly remember moments where fun changed, but rather than this being a change in my tastes or desires, it was imposed by my own sense of self-consciousness. On one occasion, when I was about 12, I remember building a wall of sand to try and repel the incoming tide on a beach. It was quite a complex structure with a main wall facing the sea and subsidiary walls and moats to direct the sea away from the further extremes of the wall. It had a series of standing stones leading away from the front down towards the water—the thinking being that I could chart the progress of the tide towards my fortress by the sequential toppling of the stones. I had spent a good while on the wall, and wall building at the beach was something that I was particularly fond of. However, on this particular day I noticed a couple of other children who looked about my age, maybe older, watching me. Although I wasn't absolutely sure, I got the sense that they were laughing at me. I remember feeling increasingly foolish—and sick. The thought that these children might think that I was playing like a small child was horrific to me, and so despite loving building walls against the sea, I climbed out from behind it and sheepishly went back to where the rest of my family were sitting. I didn't really play wall building at the beach throughout the rest of my childhood. In conversation with others I know that mine is not an isolated experience—whilst the specifics may differ the journeys away from our childhoods are markedly similar.

We have very clear structural indicators of our stages of life. Institutions mark our lives in years and the number of years we are trigger rights or expectations, privileges or responsibilities. An obvious one of these indicators in relation to ideas of fun, for many young people in the UK at least, is the ability to buy alcohol.

As a teenager the introduction of alcohol and then pubs became increasingly important to how my friends and I framed fun. Particularly from the age of about 17, fun was supposed to be synonymous with 'going out' though, in practice, going out was never nearly as much fun as it was supposed to be or as much fun as we told other people it was. My sense is that teenage years are fraught with anxieties that are unique to it. The desire to not be a child is strong for many teenagers and as our sense of fun is fermented in childhood, it is important for teenagers to attempt to forge new ways of having fun that speak to an emerging adult identity.

However, it is a relatively common experience for teenagers to put a lot of pressure on the things that are *supposed* to be fun at that age and neglect things that they as children had found fun. To a certain extent we recapture this childish sensibility as we become more confident in our adult selves—but by this time we have lost much of the capacity to experience fun in the way that we did as children.

When I think about how I have fun these days, it is a mixture of feeling liberated from responsibility, and also an absence of anxiety, and a more vicarious fun experienced particularly through my children. These run alongside the break from normalcy. Holidays have increased in importance from my twenties where the time away from routines and the possibility of a more relaxed or spontaneous attitude to the day ahead has become precious. I think that moments of euphoria have also become increasingly important to me—laughing uncontrollably, marvelling at a view and dancing are all things that are discernible and fun. There are things that I have found consistently fun in the last few years and I associate with the more euphoric feelings and an intense form of fun. I have also found that a shedding of inhibitions allows for increased fun. An occasion that springs to mind was at a music festival in the summer of 2015. My partner, a close friend and I spent an afternoon outside of our tents getting dressed up for an evening exploring the festival site. It was our friend's birthday and all three of us were in a buoyant mood and drank and danced from the early evening to late at night. There were moments of euphoria when we looked around and were aware that we were having great fun—as opposed to being distracted away from recognising fun in the moment, the recognition of fun was part of the fun. The huge numbers of people dancing, jumping, smiling and laughing with each other accentuated the centrality of sociality to fun. There were many occasions throughout the evening where the three of us looked at each other, affirming the fun that we were all experiencing.

Whilst I have fun in less contrived surroundings than the one just described, there is an interesting dichotomy between how we imagine ourselves as increasingly sophisticated over time and the desire to have experiences free from inhibition, sanction and self-consciousness—a return to our relationship to the world when we are children.

Before talking specifically about experiences of fun in adulthood and the consequent interpretation of behaviour I want to spend some time outlining how we come to imagine childhood and adulthood as distinct, and to think about the processes of transition that are assumed to occur between apparently distinct stages of the life course. This is important for then understanding the ambiguous relationship that adults have with fun as well as societal expectations of appropriate and inappropriate fun making.

Transitions and the Life Course

The separation between stages of our lives is contextually bound and relatively arbitrary. There is no a-cultural journey from childhood to adulthood and each society organises transitions in ways that make sense to them. Here fun in adulthood is examined with reference to transitions from childhood and adolescence as they are generally understood in twenty-first-century Europe. The life course is fairly uniformly understood in the West as generally referring

> to the interweave of age-graded trajectories, such as work careers and family pathways, that are subject to changing conditions and future options, and to short term transitions ranging from school leaving to retirement. (Elder 1994: 5)

As such everyone acknowledges, for whatever reason, when a transition from youth to adulthood occurs. What is interesting for the study of fun are assumptions that are made about the depth of change that occurs in this transition. We tend to imagine that there are profound differences between children and adults, but at the same time insist that there is some sort of persistent personality that underpins each individual. This chimes with our characterisation of childish fun as distinct from adult fun in the construction of these two stages of the life course whilst at the same time acknowledging that individuals have fun in ways that transcend these distinctions. For example, I have loved football in a similar way throughout my childhood, adolescence and adulthood. This is also true of riding bicycles, jumping off rocks into the sea and making a mess thinking that I might not have to clear it up.

Becker and Situational Adjustments

In an article in 1964 Howard Becker discusses this apparent contradiction. In 'Personal Change in Adult Life' he makes the observation that we think of ourselves as 'governed by deep and relatively unchanging components of personality or self' (Becker 1964: 40) whilst at the same time suggesting, from Brim, that there are no personality traits that persist across 'any and all situations and social roles' (Becker 1964: 40). Becker reconciles these apparently contradictory positions in what he calls 'situational adjustments'. Taking the classic symbolic interactionist stance he simply suggests that 'individuals take on the characteristics required by the situation they participate in' (Becker 1964: 41). It is this that provides what Becker refers to as a 'wedge' to prise open the problem of change in adulthood whilst at the same time recognising coherence of personality between stages of the life course. He suggests that in the situational adjustments that we make, modifying elements of personality and behaviour to suit particular contexts, we are also engaged in a process of commitment where 'externally unrelated interests of the person become linked in such a way as to constrain future behaviour'. For Becker this 'suggests an approach to the problem of personal stability in the face of changing situations' (Becker 1964: 41). In other words, these are the social and personal forces which, to an extent, determine who we think we are and how we think people like us should behave. These forces act as the mediators of coherence in behaviour, despite changes in the contexts within which we find ourselves. When it comes to fun then, a person will recognise that an adult like them will *not* have fun in the same way as they did when they were a child *until* very specific circumstances permit that behaviour in a way that marries the changing context with the a coherent personality. An example of this is when parents or grandparents are permitted to enjoy 'childish' fun, but only when they are with their children or grandchildren. So for Becker it is in the context in which personality happens that there is change. In fact, he goes as far to suggest that 'personality changes' are often 'present only in the eye of the beholder' (Becker 1964: 41). The ways in which assumptions about change are reached are for Becker 'excessively parochial' as they are always reached from an adult point of view. So the transition from childhood through adolescence is viewed retrospectively by people—adults—who assume they no longer have a deep connection to the condition that they themselves have defined as distinct. Rather playfully Becker muses 'what would our theories look like if we made greater effort to capture the child's point of view?' (Becker 1964: 44). As the belief in change is so widespread and uniform, Becker suggests that situational adjustment is frequently a collective process, and the collective can be small, such as a group of individuals, or huge, such as a society. It is important to recognise the process of situational adjustment when it comes to accounting for why we tend to behave and react in similar ways to similar phenomena, particularly when it comes to something like age appropriateness and fun:

> A structural explanation of personal change has important implications for attempts to deliberately mould human behaviour. In particular, it suggests that we need not try to develop deep and lasting interests, be they values or personality traits, in order to produce the behaviour that we want. It is enough to create situations which will coerce people into behaving as we want them to create the conditions under which other rewards will become linked to continuing this behaviour. (Becker 1964: 52–3)

For fun this reward process involves social legitimation—being taken seriously, having gravitas and a degree of authority or power. Interestingly, this looks as though it stands in contrast to the 'fun morality' outlined by Martha Wolfenstein, where social legitimacy in the 1950s, particularly for mothers, was to demonstrate how much fun you could have. However, this is perhaps an example of the situational adjustment that Becker is talking about where, collectively, a principle that may or may not relate to individual personal characteristics becomes important and is then responded to.

The separation of childhood and adulthood marks a rite of passage from a notional lack of responsibility but a marked lack of status in childhood to responsibility and an increase in status in adulthood. Indeed, Neugarten, Moore and Lowe claim 'in all societies, age is one of the bases for the ascription of status and one of the underlying dimensions by which social interaction is regulated' (Neugarten et al. 1965: 710). It is therefore important for the maintenance of established power dynamics between generations that we recognise distinct phases of life and then accord those phases distinct privileges. So important is it that these phases are recognised they have been practically formalised. So, as early as 1965 Neugarten et al. were suggesting that there is a 'prescriptive timetable' that orders major life events (Neaugarten et al. 1965: 711). Accordingly, norms and expectations of how successful/unsuccessful, conventional/unconventional a life is can be judged against this timetable. With the situational adjustments that are made as a result of the prescriptive timetable we end up with an idea of age appropriateness that largely directs behaviour. When thinking about examples of how judgements become manifest, a number of phrases occurred to me, and I think they will be familiar to anybody that has grown up in the Anglophonic world. 'He's too old to be working so hard', 'she's too young/old to be wearing that style of clothing', 'that's a strange thing for a person of their age to say' are examples, and perhaps the most familiar of all 'act your age'—a statement that is deployed to regulate the behaviour of both adults and children alike. As Neugarten et al. go on to suggest:

> Personal belief in the relevance of social norms increases through the adult life span and that, in this instance as the individual ages he [sic] becomes increasingly aware of age discrimination in adult behaviour and of the system of social sanctions that operate with regard to age appropriateness. (Neugarten et al. 1965: 716)

Our transitions between distinct stages of life is institutionally marked, particularly in wealthier parts of the world. It is clear to a population that they have moved from primary education to secondary education, for example. This is normally indicated by young people being moved from one building to a completely different building. We expect then these youngsters to rebuild relationships with others in relation to the new set of expectations that we have of them that are pegged to this new institutional affiliation—the secondary school. In the UK, there is another shift from 16 years old and yet another at 18. This clear demarcation of particular stages of the life course mean that it is inevitable that something happens to our view of ourselves and what is appropriate at any particular point in our lives (Elder 1994; Oesterle et al. 2004; Fincham et al. 2011; Bengtson et al. 2012). The delineation of life into discrete stages has a profound effect on how we behave and feel.

For whatever reason, we also appear to follow fairly uniform patterns of well-being and happiness according to this prescriptive timetable. The Office for National Statistics has monitored reported well-being of a sample of the UK population for a number of years. As Fig. 4.1 illustrates, there appears to be a U-shaped relationship between whether a person reported levels of satisfaction with their life, whether they felt that their lives were worthwhile and whether they reported being happy yesterday.

Younger and older people reported higher levels on all three of these scales and people in their thirties, forties or fifties reported lower levels. This reflects an established narrative of increasing responsibility and anxiety throughout adult life that seems to peak in middle age and then recedes, particularly after retirement.

When this appears to be so uniformly experienced it is strange that we don't really do anything to mediate the effects of this negative consequence of organising stages of life as we do. Fun and playfulness, at whatever stage of life, is understood to relieve us from anxiety or distract us from the things that are making us unhappy—and in childhood fun is an important element in a positive experience of it. As was explained in the chapter on theorising fun, the temporal element is important for distinguishing fun from other affective responses to stuff, but one of the frequently reported negative effects of getting older is not having time to do what you want. It strikes me that one corrosive effect of pinning appropriate behaviour to particular stages of life is what happens to fun.

Adolescence, Well-being and Fun

As was explained in the previous chapter, childhood is particularly important for crystallising fun as a coherent phenomenon. It is also where we are first sensitised to the social requirement for it to be channelled and controlled, but also the personal realisation that part of what makes some things fun is the subversive element to some activities. In the UK at least the journey from early childhood to adulthood is dominated by schooling. From the age of about 4 until either 16 or 18 young people are subject to particular forms of pedagogic philosophy formulated to best encourage and exploit the incredible capacity for learning of young

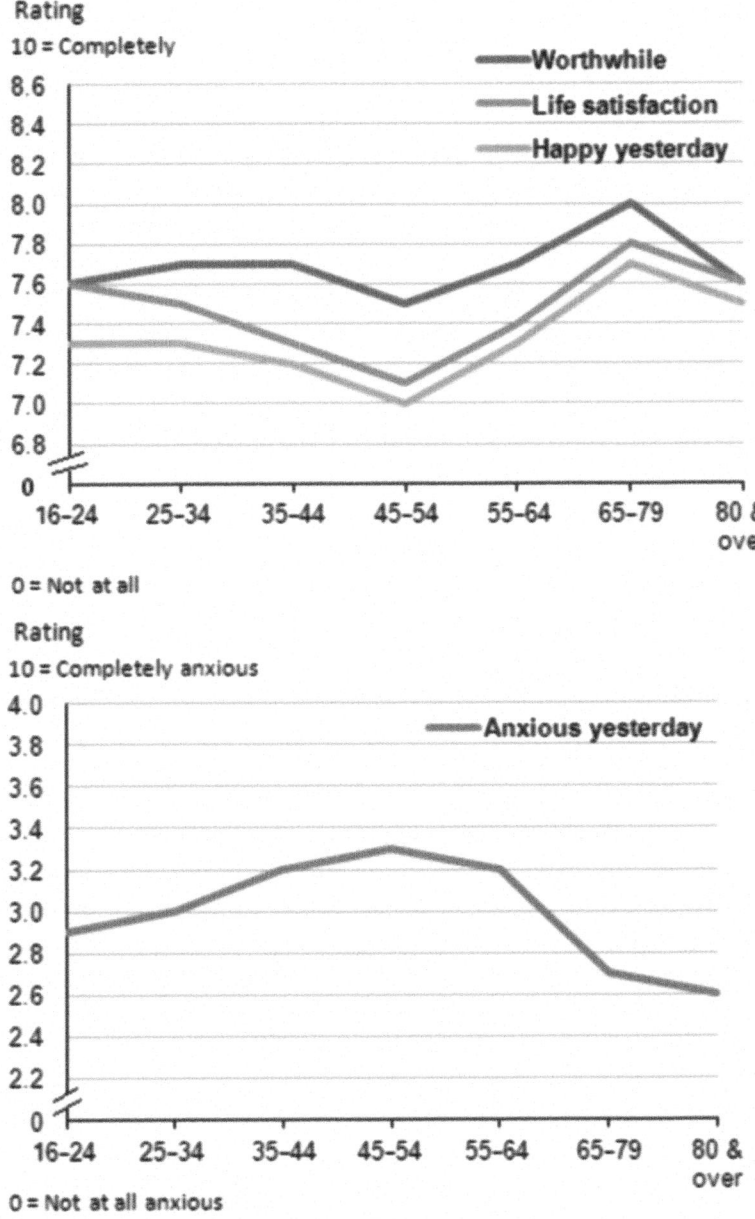

Fig. 4.1 Average personal wellbeing by age group UK 2012–13 (Office for National Statistics 2013: 14 http://www.ons.gov.uk/ons/dcp171778_319478.pdf) Licence: http://www.nationalarchives.gov.uk/doc/open-government-licence/version/3/

human beings. But what of fun in learning? In the earliest years, fun is thought to be an important tool for children's learning. Children are encouraged to have fun, explore and find out ways of doing for themselves. In early years schooling there is plenty of time in the school day that is given over to pratting about. Time for playing, and creative fun, are key building blocks in UK children's inculcation into formal, institutionalised learning. Then, year on year, the fun is squeezed out. Rules and increasingly regulated forms of pedagogy are privileged. Playtimes become shorter and less frequent between stages of schooling and the concentration on fun and joy has all but disappeared for the 15-year-old school pupils in the UK. This begs the question, why do we think that fun and self-expression are so valuable for learning—at a stage when our brains are at their most able to learn—but less and less valuable as we travel through schooling into adulthood?

As was discussed in the previous chapter this is a perplexing question. Plenty of scholars of young people point out the role of adolescence in the 'adult in waiting' discourse mooted by Aries (1962) and perhaps this offers clues as to why fun is drained out of our childhood as we head towards adulthood. For example, Johnson, Crosnoe and Elder argue that adolescence is a period for translating childhood experiences into 'competencies and statuses' that are then used in the transition to adulthood (Johnson et al. 2011: 273). This positions teenage years as a key transitionary phase in life with distinct and isolated features, and whilst it certainly feels like this when you are in the midst of it, it is difficult to know quite how much of our adolescence is distinct from the rest of our lives outside of informal and formal framing of experiences as adolescent. The disappearance of a fun that is understood of as childish or innocent to be replaced by a more knowing and perhaps less innocent model of fun is a common experience. We seem to be aware that this happens and are not happy about it but seem powerless to prevent it.

The process of responding to external pressures in determining the fun that we feel able to have is almost universally experienced—tales of the regrets of adults on the passing of childhood but there is little or no discussion of how enjoyment or pleasure, let alone fun, is translated from childhood to adulthood.

Fun in Adulthood

When we think about fun in relation to adults we often refer back to childhood. When adults are reported to have fun, it is very often resonant of non-adult behaviour and is clearly associated with times when the norms of expected behaviour are not applied or not adhered to.

Ian Wellard confronts this problem in his book *Sport, Fun and Enjoyment* (Wellard 2013). In it Wellard recognises that fun, enjoyment and pleasure are essential for continued participation in sport and says 'the accounts provided by the children and adults in this book clearly demonstrate that their experiences of sport could not be fully explained as "just" fun' (Wellard 2013: 120). The problem here, however, is that he then goes on to say 'in doing so, their descriptions of how their experiences were fun for a range of contrasting reasons bear testament to claims that fun and enjoyment are significant aspects for taking part and for future enjoyment' (Wellard 2013: 120). This perhaps relates to the observation made by Blythe and Hassenzahl about commitment—or the lack of commitment—when it comes to fun. I am sure that Wellard is correct that fun alone is not enough for continued participation in sport but the conflation with enjoyment blurs the line between what exactly is being referred to in this quote—fun or fun *and* enjoyment. It also conflates adults and children by deploying words that are normally associated with either to varying degrees. If you are talking only about children it might seem reasonable to suggest that fun is enough for the continued participation of many children in sport—in fact, if I think about Sunday morning football, it seems reasonable to suggest that it is enough for some adults.

The association with a lack of seriousness, frivolity and the levity of fun does not sit comfortably with the sorts of ways in which adulthood is defined through norms established through the life course. These norms are related to ideas of responsibility and irresponsibility—and fun is associated with a lack of responsibility. This contradicts a discourse of responsibility and of what it is to be a good adult. It is little wonder then that many adults have an ambiguous relationship with fun. This is also why not behaving as we are supposed to or as we normally do is a basis for fun in adulthood.

How Do Adults Have Fun?

This does beg the question, how do adults have fun? The extracts from the survey that make up the next section of this chapter point towards two key orientations to fun that relate to fun in childhood. The first is that other people remain important—fun as a socially manifest phenomenon is reinforced—and the other is that the process of inhibition that was illustrated is expressed in the data about adult fun. Either the fun that is professed is fairly restrained, that is, it doesn't involve an unknowing abandonment of childhood fun, or it is intentionally disinhibited, involving specific occasions or, for quite a few UK participants alcohol, again distinct from the disinhibition of childhood.

Something happens in the transition between childhood and adulthood, normally the earlier teenage years, where fun is desired under the conditions that it was experienced as a child, but is increasingly inhibited by the norms of adulthood. Younger teenagers are in the ambiguous position of wanting both childish fun and adulthood but not being able to fully realise either. As we move into adulthood, we loosen the desire for childish fun for the most part—despite what people say—and then take fun in the rarified or refined world of adult pleasures or the more raucous and transgressive world of adult fun. We also develop a sense of vicarious fun. This form of fun is most commonly expressed through the identification with fun in time spent with children. So rather than enjoying the childish fun ourselves we have fun being involved with children having childish fun. When talking to adults about fun it appears to become apparent that there is a distinction between those who have their own children or grandchildren and those that do not when it comes to vicarious fun. The instances of people mentioning fun through others, particularly children, is pronounced for parents and grandparents. Of course, this is primarily because of the opportunities for contact with children there are for parents and grandparents and also, for many, the reduced opportunities parenthood offers for sustained time away from children. The distinction between people in terms of their experiences of vicarious fun are not to do with the type of person one is, but more the opportunities a person has to have fun where the enjoyment of others—particularly children—is not a prerequisite for their own fun.

Distinction Between Spaces Designated for Fun and Fun in Other Spaces

Adults have quite a linear relationship to space and fun. Spaces are designed for fun or not fun—and the types of fun that we have in them depend on their functional relationship to fun. For example, a nightclub has an overt and clear fun utility. Fun revolving around drinking alcohol and dancing is sanctioned and designed for. It would not be appropriate to behave in a library at 2.30 in the afternoon as if having fun in a nightclub. The examples of workplaces that are designed for a looser relationship to control also have areas designated for productivity, for example, desks, creative hubs, and areas for 'fun', for example, slides, table football, basketball courts. On a broader scale, buildings and public space have very specific utilities. The spaces that we live in are normally clearly demarcated as being for a specific type of experience or experiences. As adults we are finely tuned to recognise the tenor or atmosphere of a space, even if its utility is not immediately apparent. We will seek out the space that best suits the atmosphere that we require. When it comes to fun, adults are generally able to discern what they need to satisfy a particular orientation to fun at any given time—what props will be needed (alcohol, an activity, food, etc.) and what mood is desired. This is indicative of the compartmentalisation of fun that happens in the journey from childhood to adulthood. This demarcation of space is less apparent to younger people who are then schooled through a variety of methods into understanding appropriate behaviour in different spaces. Fun in spaces not designed for fun appeals to the more transgressive or rebellious side of fun—and sometimes requires a degree of disinhibition, again something associated more with children than adults. As will be demonstrated, most of the fun reported to me in the course of the fun survey adhered to the rules of space, unless there was a knowing transgression

Adults Having Fun

This section of the chapter deals directly with adults' recent experiences of fun. As part of the survey conducted into fun in the spring and summer of 2014 respondents were asked to describe, in as much detail as they wished, a recent occasion where they had fun. The results were fascinating, particularly when set alongside the answers to questions about fun in childhood.

As with the other chapters that involve data from the survey conducted as part of this project, there is a large amount of overlap in the coded data. When a respondent says that they had fun when they went to a pub with a friend and their sister, ended up getting drunk and then unexpectedly went on for a dance at a club the coding for that data would involve 'friends', 'family', 'pub', 'drinking', 'clubbing', 'dancing' and 'spontaneity'. Each of these discrete categories appears in the presentation of the data and I have chosen where and when to use direct quotes to illustrate the themes that emerged in the data. A particular feature of the responses to this section of the survey was the length of the answers—they were very brief. Unlike the relatively lengthy stories offered in the section on childhood it seemed to me that there was a 'taken for grantedness' that the situations described are fun. What is interesting, however, is that there was a degree of uniformity in the testimonies, there is not as much as in the much longer stories of fun in childhood.

Other People

Given the social nature of fun it is unsurprising to find that other people feature largely in the accounts of fun provided for the survey. Whilst it is clear that there were many more instances where fun was had with other people than I have counted I decided that I would code to other people only when they were specified. The reason for this is that I think that it indicates that the people are at the forefront of the memory of the fun that was had.

Other People: Friends

By quite some distance, friends featured most prominently in the examples of recent fun that the adult respondents shared. The situations described were many and varied, but the importance of friends to having fun is clear. Some accounts were very general:

> Hanging out with friends. Talking. Chatting. Eating. Drinking. Watching films. Eating out. (F41, No specified occupation)

Whilst there are no specific incidents cited here, there is acknowledgement that the relationships between friends are productive in terms of fun. It is the friend relationship that often establishes the context in which fun can occur, but also generates the fun in the moment. In these circumstances it has a totalising effect in the interpretation of the experience. People understand that they have fun with friends—this is a context—and this orientation to experiences with friends opens the space for *having* fun. This highlights the relational component of fun. Orientation to relationships is crucial to having this sort of fun. A distinct feature of close relationships is that of trust. It is clear from other parts of the study of fun that being in situations where a person can relax, be free from current concerns, feel able to let themselves go is important. There were stories that were suffused with the sort of close warmth that comes from trusting friend relationships. A paralegal practitioner from London said:

> I spent a weekend in London with my best friend (from Uni). We went to a bar (which we have visited before) on Friday night, and on Saturday (slightly hungover), we spent the day in London having lunch with another friend (also from Uni), who had travelled down from Manchester. We spent the majority of the afternoon eating a nice meal and lots of cake. Then we went for a walk in sunny Regent's Park. Discussion was mainly current updates on how we were, reminiscing about old times and being updated on how others from Uni were doing. (F25, Paralegal)

A similar situation was described by a 22-year-old in Brighton:

> A few weeks ago I saw a few old friends whom I hadn't seen properly for a couple of years. We sat in the bedroom of one of the friends and stayed up until the small hours catching up and drinking. We played PS3 and watched a few Youtube gems, too, but it was mostly just talking and joking around. (M22, Student)

In both of these excerpts there is a sense of ease with the people with whom the respondents are having fun that underpins the experiences or events described. Drinking alcohol will be discussed in more detail a little later on, but it is interesting that both of the previous stories also involved a degree of drinking, as well as reminiscence. Similar to the previous comment a Sales Assistant highlighted how relatively unspectacular occasions are made fun by the presence of friends:

> My fiancé's birthday, we had a friend over and we played computer games, chatted and generally it was a lot of fun without doing an awful lot. (F24, Sales assistant)

Others talked about less mundane activities involving friends:

> Last summer I went on a camping trip with two friends, and we had such fun—we swam in the sea, we hitch-hiked (my first time ever!), we camped in farmers' fields, we bought delicious food and had camp fires—it was just a whole week of glorious fun! (F33, PhD student)

There were a few people that highlighted the ways in which fun could be had with friends even if elements of the experience do not immediately appear as fun. In the next excerpt a student describes a discussion where the subject matter did not detract from the fun inherent in spending time with her friend:

> Yesterday was one of the best days of my life. I had breakfast at a nice new café with a friend. Then I went to Taj. Then I went to a clothes swap at a friend's house. I got quite a few nice new pieces of clothing and chatted about fun stuff but also about rape and abusive relationships. (F28, Student)

As will be seen, many of the responses that I will use to illustrate other aspects of adults' orientations to fun involve friends, in fact 40% of the responses to the question 'tell me about a recent occasion where you had fun' explicitly mentioned friends. It is fair to assume that when a person has said something like 'playing snooker' (M41, Senior research fellow), they were playing with friends.

Other People: Family

Many people explicitly referred to family members when recalling a recent occasion of fun (18%). Whilst this is not nearly as many as mentioned family in stories of fun in childhood, it is still a sizable proportion of the respondents given the relative overall lack of uniformity in the responses. Perhaps predictably many parents of younger children mentioned them as central to stories of having fun. There were several people that gave brief accounts of time with their kids. An occupational therapist in Nottingham said:

> Today with my children, climbing a big hill and being outdoors in the countryside. (F36, Occupational therapist)

Whilst a lecturer in the Midlands said:

> Playing rounders in the park with my kids. (F43, Lecturer)

The importance of wider family setting the context for having fun with kids was highlighted by a number of people:

> Last week when we took the kids to Aviemore and were going down the water slide in the swimming pool. Also at my brother's BBQ on Saturday when we were shooting an airgun at targets. (F36, Researcher)

In this extract the fun activities are done with the children, but the site of some of the fun was at a brother's house. It was often the case that fun with family was a question of hosting—where a party or barbecue was being held. This is similar to the narratives of fun in childhood, where the family, particularly during holidays, is the locus for having fun. It was not just young children that were cited as being people to have fun with:

> Going to a club with my eldest daughter and her friend, it was gypsy punk music, burlesque, acrobats, face painting, storytelling, circus acts and lots of topless women and no pervs. (F47, unemployed)

This is an interesting account for all sorts of reasons. Aside from involving a family member it also speaks to ideas of disinhibition and transgression. There is a tacit acknowledgement that this environment is one that can be interpreted as transgressive in a way that the author does not want when she says that there were 'no pervs'. A less dramatic response was provided by a parent from Southend, who said:

> Of an evening when my adult sons, partner and I get back in from work we generally eat dinner watching 'pointless' on the TV. I love the conversation and banter, the laughing and the piss taking as we watch the TV and eat some food. (F52, No work specified)

The changing nature of child/parent relationship is accentuated in the previous quotes, but the relationship is still one that has the potential to provide the conditions for fun. In a similar way to friends, the closeness of good familial relations accentuates the potential for having fun. Trust, familiarity and, to certain extent, repetition are features of fun borne out of relationships in which people feel secure. Siblings were mentioned, as were grandparents, grandchildren and cousins.

Other People: Partner

As with friends it is clear that there were many stories of fun where partners were present but are not specified in the submission. That said, I was still surprised that partners were not more frequently mentioned (6%). In fact, it tended to be younger respondents that mentioned partners. There were several occasions where partner's birthdays were mentioned, a typical example being:

> My girlfriend's birthday party, everyone was dressed up, everyone was cool, friendly, drunk, sociable. (M32, Student)

There were other people that specified their partner amongst friends, and that the presence of a partner augmented the fun. The next quote also indicates a lack of specific plan that underpinned many of the accounts of fun. This is despite spontaneity being surprisingly absent in words that people used to describe the situations that they found themselves in. Once again this might just be a result of the way the question was interpreted but I was still perplexed by its absence:

> [my] Boyfriend came down to my place for the weekend and we went to Preston Park in Brighton with my flatmates, kicked and threw a ball around. Went back home and had a BBQ, had a few drinks and played card games and charades. (F19, Student)

The closeness of relationships—particularly involving trust and letting go—has been highlighted as important with friends and family, and for a couple of people, this was particularly important when it came to partners. For this student from Brighton, the fun was accentuated by the alleviation offered from something troubling by a partner, who responded to the problem and then was instrumental in diverting attention away from it:

> A couple of days ago—on Brighton beach with my boyfriend. I was having a dilemma and was feeling sad about it... so we went for a walk along the beach and spent some money we don't have on fish and chips and then ice cream. We mucked about and played together and both spent lots of the day laughing! (F23, Student)

Whilst not talking about a recent occasion of having fun, a researcher from Leicester pointed out the social aspect fun—but was also clear about their partner as instrumental to this social experience, and for her spending time with her partner is associated in her mind with having fun.

> It still remains a very much social activity for me. Now fun is spending time with my partner or with friends travelling, going out, spending time with them. (F30, Researcher)

The importance of the social in having fun cannot be overstated. However, for some there is a degree of closeness and trust in certain relationships that permits a certain type of activity to become defined as fun—even to the extent that just being around certain people is described by some as fun.

Intimacy

Whilst some of the experiences or relationships in the previous section could be described as intimate I have decided to reserve the word to describe situations that involve a degree of intimacy that indicates a freedom within a relationship that is absent from other relationships. It is interesting that only one person mentioned sex when it came to a recent experience of fun. Whilst you might not anticipate that many people would want to talk about sex in a survey, it was anonymous, and given that sex and fun are often assumed to be synonymous in the popular imagination I thought that at least a couple more people would have mentioned it. The lack of references to it supports the assertion made later in the book that certain phenomena being described as fun are less a description of our experience of them and more a discursive construction of how we wish activities to be understood and communicated. Subsequently this is inflected onto our sense of ourselves and sense of others. An administrator in Leeds said:

> My most recent experience of fun would be tickling my husband before bed. (F33, Administrator)

Also in the bedroom a facilities co-ordinator from Bristol talked about pants:

> This morning, doing the pants dance for my fiance while he's still in bed, I dance around getting ready whilst he sings pants, pants, pants, pants. (F33, Facilities co-ordinator)

The only person to specifically mention sex was a police officer from Hull, and even then he was a little coy about it—preferring to move on to talking about playing with his child:

> Sex related stuff recently. Or playing with my 20 month old child. He's hilarious. (M35, Police officer)

I suppose a more accurate way of describing the experiences noted above might be 'in the bedroom', but this is a space inherently associated with heightened intimacy, so I don't feel too bad about it.

Other People: Strangers

A few people (3%) mentioned strangers in their stories of recent fun, but this was in the context of either becoming friends or having a friendly experience. It was connectivity between people that did not know each other so well—alongside the experience—that was fun. A student talked about getting to know a group of people:

> I went out to the Mesmerist [pub/club] last night with my housemates' work friends, made friends with them, and drank a lot of vodka cranberry and danced to 50s music. (F20, Student)

Whilst an artists' model spoke about getting to know one person:

> I went on a date with an immensely hot girl who paid for all my drinks and kissed me with meaning. (F19, Artists' model)

However, it is the dynamic between people that creates the conditions for having fun. A chef from Glasgow made this point:

> A hiking trip up north with a bunch of strangers. The right blend of people can make anything fun I suppose. (M29, Chef)

In these data the social aspect of fun is clear. This is a phenomenon that people have with each other—and strengthens the social bonds between people. It is difficult to envisage a friendship or partnership where fun is absent. However, the way sociability and fun works changes through the life course. The transition from childhood to adulthood, at least looking at these data, is marked by a diversification of the people that we understand ourselves to have fun with—in the childhood data family featured much more heavily, for example. There are a couple of reasons for this. The first is that we become used to having positive experiences with a wider range of people—for a start we meet more and more people as life goes on—but also as the opportunities for having fun become increasingly restricted (see Chap. 3) we grab it when we can or engineer situations where fun looks likely. This is completely different from childhood where situations or opportunities are manufactured for us (playtime, school, holidays, 'play-dates', etc.)—whether we take them or not is another matter (see data in Chap. 3). The second is the point made in Chap. 2, 'Theorising Fun', where the discourse of fun—and how we make sense of fun in childhood—is far more formulaic than it is in an adult present. It is bound up with ideas of what childhood is supposed to consist of—allied to what fun is supposed to consist of—and how we communicate our experience of it to others. This touches on questions of identity—what we appear to enjoy says something about who we are. Stories of fun in childhood provide historical perspectives which are then amplified through stories in the present.

Outdoors

The next most prolific feature of the data gathered in response to the question 'tell me a recent occasion where you had fun' was stories that involved being outdoors (21%). There was a large crossover with stories of holidays, and they will be addressed more specifically a little later on. I enjoyed these stories particularly. They were suffused with a sense of joy in what Merleau-Ponty would call 'being-in-the-world' (Merleau-Ponty 2002). There was the PhD student from Manchester quoted earlier who recounted the new experiences she had whilst camping with friends, eating food and lighting fires. As with practically all of the stories, there are crossovers in the themes that are touched on here and all of these features of this time stuck in her mind and helped frame the experience as fun. It is not that one element is inherently fun but all of the elements together produce the overall experience.

A researcher from Edinburgh spoke about the importance of nature in her recent experience of fun:

> I have fun quite often when I go climbing. My holidays are great, always abroad in the sun climbing away and relaxing in the sun, in the middle of the forest with only nature around. (F39, Researcher)

The combination of being active, being on holiday and being outdoors in nature produces fun for this researcher. It is interesting to note that climbing can be quite a solitary pursuit, and this person did not mention anybody else. A TV producer from Cardiff talked about cycling in the countryside. Again, this is sometimes a solitary activity, but he also mentioned having amiable conversations with strangers as part of his recent fun:

> I cycled from a cottage in Pembrokeshire along the coast to the village of Little Haven. I'd visited my sister there on her summer holiday so sent her a photo. Had a nice chat with some old blokes over a coffee in the sun and rode back on roads I didn't know at a leisurely pace. Smashing. (M44, Television producer)

The role of the weather was also important to many people in their recent experiences of fun; 6% of respondents mentioned sunshine, possibly a consequence of the timing of the questionnaire, but it is the case that with water and beaches enjoyment is mediated by good weather.

Talking

In contrast to the stories of childhood, there were many occasions where talking or chatting was associated with fun for adults. This more sedentary experience appears to develop over the life course. Fun in childhood was not associated with simply talking—although as is suggested in a paper by Broner and Torone (2001) children do have fun with wordplay—in adulthood talking takes on a different complexion. Chatting, banter and catching up in particular were given as recent examples where people had fun. The lack of drama or event in some of these stories was nice. This speaks to the unspectacular ways in which we have fun. It is not necessarily associated with exceptional activities, but is embedded into our everyday experiences—lifting some of them from the mundane to the memorable.

> Having a long weekend in Dorset with old friends and their children this weekend. I enjoyed the things that we did together, but in terms of fun primarily enjoyed catching up and laughing together. (F36, Teacher)

Again, the fun for this person is derived from 'catching up' and 'laughing together' rather than the activities that supported or surrounded the chat. A shop assistant also talked about a period away from home with friends, but also the excitement of talking with others about politics.

> Chatting about politics with a bunch of lefties in Ullapool, with whisky, mountains, good music. Cracking. Fun because the independence campaign is so exciting and politics has been so revived and I genuinely relish the opportunity to hear people's ideas and talk to them about mine, it is 'fun' for me. (O25, Shop assistant)

The fact that this might not be everybody's cup of tea highlights the relationship between a general sense that some things can be fun, chatting, for example, and then the specifics of what individuals have fun chatting about, politics, for example.

Laughter

Often related to talking is laughter. However, when it comes to laughing related to fun it appears that discourse is an important facilitator—it was referred to as part of the fun a couple of times, but more usually it was used as a mechanism for communicating that an occasion or time was fun. Laughter was identified in very specific incidents. In response to the request to tell me about a recent experience of fun a lecturer said:

> Laughing and couldn't stop when my partner told me a story of when someone got her name wrong (doesn't sound funny but it was) and dancing crazy around my office to the 'Happy' song for no reason whatsoever. (F47, Lecturer)

But also as part of the ambience of a period of time. People identified times where they recalled laughing lots:

> When I went with my boyfriend to a very beautiful coastal town and spent two days exploring the coastline with lots of conversation/laughter. (F34, Lecturer)

People also used the term 'a real laugh' or 'a right laugh'. In my experience this is a literal term. When occasions are described as 'a laugh' it is almost always because the people involved were laughing lots:

> I went to the pub with two work colleagues, it was a real laugh. I went for a walk along the river with my husband and the dog and that was great, too. (F47, College lecturer)

There were others that talked about hilarity implying that laughter was an important component of the experience.

> I recently went out with a couple of friends for lunch. It was great to catch up with them and, conversation-wise, it was pretty hilarious. So I'd say that was pretty fun. (F18, Student)

The importance of laughter to fun is often taken for granted and assumed. However, as many of the people in this study have shown, it is not a prerequisite. That said, when it happens laughter is more often than not associated with fun. Laughter and fun share an important feature in common, making it easy to presume that they are mutually inclusive, namely, that they are both specifically temporally bound. Both start and finish at identifiable points in time. Also, they are both obvious markers of knowing that you've had a good time.

Alcohol

A consequence of the majority of responses coming from the UK is that alcohol featured heavily in the stories of recent fun. For this study about a quarter of the stories involved alcohol in some way. Rather than suggesting that this is a result of 'Broken Britain' or anything crass like that, I think that this is more a reflection of two things. The first and most important is that as fun is a social activity and many adults in the UK meet and socialise in places and situations where alcohol is present, it should then be anticipated that alcohol features in many stories where the key point is the socialising. The second and more contentious is that alcohol disinhibits people. As many people identified that a lack of inhibition, or letting go, is a core component of having fun then it is unsurprising that the most prevalent artificial disinhibitor, alcohol, is frequently present when adults have fun. A young woman who works in a bar illustrated the primacy of the social interaction whilst drinking alcohol:

> Recently I had a lot of fun hanging out in the pub where I work, drinking ale on a Sunday afternoon in the sun. My boyfriend and a few friends were there, and we played guitar in the garden and laughed a lot. (F24, Bar staff)

These stories are in direct contrast to the hysterical observations of media, particularly in the UK, about the menace of alcohol. Alcohol in these stories was not used to excess, nor was it used to strip away morality or decorum—it is more of a cultural artefact of living and socialising in the UK. A textile designer in London told a story that involved many elements that appear elsewhere in the analysis—chatting, friends, pubs, sunshine and alcohol:

> One of my best friends from university came all the way from Cardiff for the weekend to hang out in London and we spent the day drinking beer in the sunshine in Brick Lane. (F23, Freelance textile designer)

There were people that highlighted the role of alcohol in parties, but also that being drunk was an important element in the fun that they described. A student in Bournemouth said:

> Going out to a club dressed up as 1920s for my housemate's birthday. Getting drunk and dancing all night. (F21, Student)

For others the location was not mentioned but the alcohol and socialising was:

> My friends and I got together to celebrate one of our friends finishing her Masters degree, and we had some drinks and chatted for hours. It was a great time. (F28, Crafter/artist)

There were also some people that simply drank at home, with others, and had a good time:

> My boyfriend and I watched 'The Hobbit 2', lots of snack food (chicken nuggets, pizza, mozzarella dippers). We drank LOTS of wine and watched both Hobbit films, which ended up being really fun and made the films hilarious! (F21, Shop assistant)

As I have suggested, the alcohol in these stories did not appear to be a manifestation of desperation or of making up for a lack of imagination, but more something that tended to be present when adults socialised.

Trips and Holidays

As with alcohol, about a quarter of respondents (27%) mentioned holidays or trips as being recent occasions that they had had fun. As with the stories in childhood, trips and holidays marked a temporary suspension of normality and subsequently a suspension of everyday travails. There were day trips with children, travels abroad, specific experiences and general observations about how holidays felt. A university professor told of a recent trip to Florida with her daughter:

> Last summer going to Disneyworld in Florida with my daughter and going to the waterparks there—we both love water—the best bit was the wave machine in the lake. Absolutely massive waves that sent you whooshing back almost all the way to the shore. We would hold hands, count it down and just get swept away—kept going back there during the trip and spent two whole days in that waterpark. (F49, Professor)

The holiday incorporates many elements found elsewhere in stories of fun. Family, water, excitement are all here. It is a nice narrative for the mixture of the general and specific. The holiday itself was fun and as way of example the respondent illustrates with the story of the wave machine. Short breaks were also mentioned, and the feeling of a suspension from normality was highlighted by an adviser:

> Girlie weekend seeing the sights in Paris—did very silly things… the funniest being a competition to see who could be photographed with the best looking person without them knowing. (F49, Adviser)

The story of friends in Paris being silly—and a bit naughty—is a particularly pertinent expression of a construction of fun that can be recognised and affirmed. In a communicative way this person is very clearly saying something about the sort of person they are, the friendships they have and, through the story of transgression, giving an indication of their idea of fun—because it is not everybody's. Being away from home permits types of behaviour distinct from behaviour at home:

> A few years ago (I hope this is recent enough!), I went to a conference in Lisbon with a number of colleagues. I was a PhD student at the time, and some of the colleagues I was with were also friends of mine. A group of us went out for a meal and then some drinks on our first night there, and much fun was had. We had far too many caipirinhas, and spent the evening telling funny stories and sharing jokes. There was a lot of laughter, and although the following morning wasn't much fun at all (!) it was probably the most fun I'd had in a while. (F31, Lecturer)

This last excerpt speaks to the point made by Podilchak when he talks of the equalisation of power relationships in having fun. Friendships are rarely predicated on formal hierarchies—even if they may appear to reflect them, unlike other areas of life and this trip abroad highlights the non-hierarchical nature of moments of fun—this can sometimes be associated with disinhibition or the loosening of formality. The consumption of caipirinhas appears to have assisted this process.

Music

Music played a role in many people's experiences of fun (17%); this included going to concerts or gigs and dancing as well as playing. Several people simply named gigs they had recently attended. One person said 'going to a Half Man Half Biscuit gig and jumping around' (M43, Social worker) and another said they 'went to see Muse last year. Much fun'

(F25, Operations manager). A mature student talked about how unexpectedly bumping into people at a gig prompted an evening that was filled with fun:

> At a gig in London—my partner and I randomly bumped into a couple we had met weeks before in Brighton... so we all hung out at the gig, and then decided to run around London and tell stories and pop into pubs. It was unexpected and a lot of fun. (F29, Student)

The gig itself is not the fun in this last excerpt, rather the site of fun—the fun was found in the interactions between the people in the story. Another great example of this was provided by a London student—but rather than attendance at an event provoking a more spontaneous fun, attendance at the event was the outcome of spontaneity:

> Met with friends for a few sociable drinks, but then unintentionally we got a little drunk and ended up going to an all night trance party at a derelict building in London. It was fun as it was not planned and happened out of the blue. (M35, Student)

It was not just listening to other musicians that was identified as fun—some people talked about their own playing—however, it was always with reference to being with others.

> I had fun at an event I sang at recently—the event itself was good but the people that I was singing with are extremely funny and we had a blast! (F49, Senior technical officer)

Nobody said they had fun making music alone:

> I went to a brilliant family band camp. I had fun catching up with old friends, meeting new ones, singing and playing my violin. (F38, Community arts worker)

The ways in which music facilitated fun was varied, but the presence of music in stories of fun suggests to me at least that many people have fun when there is music around.

Events

Related to music in some cases was the idea of fun at events or of events being fun in of themselves. Events provide the sanctioned space for fun, reflecting the idea that fun happens in sanctioned places and times, and is inappropriate in other places and times. As I have said, gigs were often mentioned:

> I went to a gig in Brighton about a week ago and I really enjoyed that. I like going to gigs and just find it a fun way to have some time off work. (F21, Student)

Another person said:

> Going to a gig for a friend's birthday in London. Was tired and not in the mood but loved it. Band were an old festival band from my 20's, 30's, danced, sang and had 'fun'. (F50, Part-time lecturer)

As with practically all of the contributions there was a social element to the fun:

> Went to see Miranda at the O2 with two of my friends. Laughed a lot and it was fun because of that plus I hadn't seen my friends in a while so it was nice to catch up. (F19, Student)

This person enjoyed the event, and may well have described it as fun if they had gone by themselves; however, it is the friends and the catching up that are important to the event as a whole being fun. A couple of people mentioned plays:

> At a friend's leaving do last weekend, we had snacks and talked then went to see a short play put on at a local college. My friend's daughter's boyfriend was in the play. (F48, Physical therapist)

Another said:

> Hmmm...fun is not so straightforward now. I guess a great night out with friends or a BBQ and beer is fun now. I recently watched Jeeves and Wooster in the West End—that was a lot of fun. (F30, Academic)

This last excerpt is interesting for the acknowledgement that having fun is more complex than it had previously been; it gets more complicated as we move through the life course.

Play and Games

There were plenty of occasions described that were playful, but about 20% of people mentioned activities that might be called play or games. Some mentioned organised games such as football or paintballing but others talked about a form of play that is more often associated with childhood. A student in Brighton said:

> Going for a walk from Falmer to Lewes, up and down the hills, sitting on the grass and enjoying the sun. Rolling down a hill, then going up and then rolling down again. (F20, Student)

This story is a nice example of doing something that directly harks back to the sort of organic fun children tend to enjoy. In another response that spoke very clearly to the data from childhood memories a 29-year-old talked about an organised but also made up game played by other adults:

> Organising and playing a mock 'Olympic Games' with friends in a local park. We competed against each other in a variety of fun events, and dressed up in the colours of the countries that we were allocated to represent. I was 29 years old. (M30, Economic researcher)

Another person talked about how children's fun was facilitated by adults, who were in turn playing:

> Piggy back races yesterday afternoon in the park—one child on each parent. (F42, University professor)

Generally speaking, there is a shift in emphasis from childhood into adulthood away from games towards less obvious, and in some senses, more passive forms of fun—drinking, talking, watching, and so on. This does not mean that fun is any less playful, just that it incorporates experiences that, as children, we do not tend to find much fun.

Active

There were also plenty of stories that spoke of a more active type of fun. These people were involved with either creative or physically specialised or demanding activities. These forms of fun tended to involve techniques or skills that take time to learn or take time to work towards. Several of these accounts involved sporting endeavours. One woman said:

> I cycled the tour of Flanders sportive. I wanted to find out whether I could ride the route the pro riders are taking including the cobbles and steep climbs. It was a marvellous day, thousands of other riders and lots of honey cake and caramel waffles were consumed. (F39, Researcher)

This wasn't just a bicycle ride—it would have taken training, high levels of fitness and a degree of competence to complete. A 66-year-old consultant from California also talked about a feat of endurance and skill that afforded him high degrees of fun:

> I just rode 5,000 miles by motorcycle from Napa to Austin Texas and back taking in some beautiful parts of the US. (M66, Consultant)

It was not just activities that extended over long periods of time that were mentioned in relation to active forms of fun. There were also those that experienced fun in a very physical sense, as was illustrated by this garden centre manager:

> Anything that involves travel is fun for me, and that includes local travel. I love seeing new places. Recently I went to Costa Rica, where I tried zip lining for the first time, across long valleys in the rain forest. I was terrified at the prospect of doing this, but determined… afterwards I grinned for hours! (F59, Garden Centre manager)

In this excerpt alongside the physically active dimension there is also the thrill of the ride on the zip wire. In fact, excitement accompanied a number of stories that involved a more physical engagement with fun. There were other activities that incorporated levels of participation in an activity requiring degrees of specialism or knowledges, as was exemplified by a retired school teacher:

> Having my god-daughter here on a visit to London, playing with my material collection, making her a top. Attending a rug making course with my friend Diane. (F71, Retired school teacher)

These accounts of fun incorporating active participation in things that involve physical expertise, skill and knowledges are interesting for the questions they raise about how the commitment to specialisms become fun at times. In Blythe and Hassenzahl's table of the distinction between fun and happiness the idea of commitment and transgression are important—and relates to the responses that carried either physically challenging or skilled elements. For them transgression and commitment sit at polar ends of a spectrum, where transgression involves rule breaking and commitment involves absorption and an acceptance of the rules around a particular activity. In the examples above there is a level of commitment that has to be present in order that the motorcycle gets ridden safely or the rug making happens. However, there can be transgressive elements discretely hidden in the committed engagement. This is a microcosmic version of the fooling about at work that Roy talks about on production lines. For Blythe and Hassenzahl attending the rug making course may well be pleasurable, but the fun starts when it goes wrong or the participants start messing about.

Children and Childishness

Surprisingly, few people mentioned either playing with children or behaving childishly. I say surprising as abstractly fun is often mentioned alongside childishness or silliness, and is associated with childhood more than adulthood. About 10% of respondents mentioned either playing with children or behaving in a childish manner. A patent attorney from Nottingham said:

> Bouncing on a trampoline at friend's house extension warming party. (F36, Patent attorney)

Whilst a student, who also worked in a shop, in Brighton talked about playing table tennis that became increasingly chaotic:

> Last Saturday me and three friends went to watch the ladies football match at the Albion. Afterwards, we randomly decided to drive to the Brighton Marina and get a McDonalds. Whilst at the Marina we discovered that there are ping pong tables that you can play for free. So we stayed there and played ping pong for about an hour. We started off playing it sensibly sticking to the actual rules. But after a while, it got a bit silly, and we were hitting the ball really hard and making it fly off in different directions to make the other players run really far to get it. We just laughed the whole time. It was nice because as we're all 3rd year students, we hadn't spent time like that together for a long time. I felt like I could just forget about my dissertation for that hour. It also felt quite child-like and silly, and we rarely get to behave like that these days. (F21, Student and sales assistant)

Alongside these acts of childishness came stories where actually playing with children was fun; a social worker describes playing with her child.

> Playing in the park today with my 2 year old, watching her giggle hysterically. (F40, Social worker)

And a teacher in Brighton said:

> Rolling around on the grass with my son. Toddlers are good at silliness and I was busy thinking of things that would make him laugh, and he was copying me. (F37, Teacher)

Whilst it is not entirely clear from these data, I think that the delineation between fun in childhood and fun in adulthood is more stark than many of us assume. The sorts of things that we experience as fun are not necessarily how we imagine fun in the abstract. Generally, it was the case that discourse becomes important in adulthood, whilst physically doing is important in childhood.

Eating and Food

It is worth mentioning eating and food as being a theme that emerged in another 10% of cases from the data. As with drinking, this is because of the opportunity food affords for socialising. This is illustrated by a 20-year-old student:

> Went for a meal for a friend's birthday. It was fun because there was a big group of us and it was good to spend time all together and talk to some of my friends who I don't spend much time with. (F20, Student)

What is interesting was the ages of people that spoke about food; they tended to be younger respondents. A 25-year-old classroom assistant said 'visiting friends at their home for Sunday lunch' (F25, Primary teaching assistant). A student said that a recent occasion of fun for him was that he 'went to my friends for a picnic in her garden' (M19, Student).

These data talk to the more sedentary fun that is sometimes associated with adulthood, and tends not to be thought of as a characteristic of fun in childhood. The fun around food and eating, also chatting, is indicative of an adult orientation to having fun.

No Fun

There were very few people that reacted negatively to the request to tell me about a recent occasion when they had fun. As would be expected, this is in contrast to the data on work, where many people struggled to identify fun; practically all of the occasions mentioned in this section of the survey happened outside of work. However, there were a couple of people that could not identify a recent occasion of fun:

> I don't have fun anymore. I have drunk weekends and fuck this shit work weeks. (No info supplied)

A proofreader said:

I don't have much fun now to be honest, but I suppose the closest I get to an experience of fun is taking my horse out for a hack and having a long canter/gallop on the sand tracks with friends and their horses. (F26, Proofreader)

And a lawyer also struggled to identify a recent occasion:

Hmmm it's been a bit fun free lately. There's been some nice [times] but no fun for over a year. Sorry! (M49, Lawyer)

There were really very few people that could not identify any recent occasion of fun in their adult lives (five in total). But, as has been mentioned I will not pretend that the data here is unbiased. It is the beginning of a discussion about fun, and the elements of social class or of health are missing. I think it is reasonable to assume that a much broader range of people would have garnered very different results. The propensity of healthy, relatively young, mostly middle class people to report levels of fun is bound to be higher than those struggling, financially, physically or socially.

Conclusions

From these data it looks as though fun becomes increasingly rarefied as we get older. In comparison with the stories from childhood we appear more inhibited, less physically active and have less of a sense of naughtiness from the tales from adulthood.

The transition from child to youth and youth to adult and the subsequent gradations of adulthood all seem to encourage the compartmentalisation of fun to ever decreasing times and spaces. In this way other forms of non-labour become important. Relaxation, for example, becomes a byword for a pleasant and distracted state where we feel unencumbered by concerns of the present—but discursively it is of a different affective order than fun. It is interesting that this sort of distinction is made between both distracted experiences as though one is more adult than the other. In conversation with a friend online I had suggested that the opportunities for having fun decrease as we get older and that you have to be either increasingly defiant in your having fun or creative. He replied by saying, 'Is fun being replaced by downtime when we're not doing all the stuff we have to, and that is enough? Fun might even be tiring.' In this statement my friend has loaded fun with tacit features that are not present in 'downtime'. For Becker this is an example of a situational adjustment, albeit underpinned with fatigue, that makes sense of a period of life where there are expectations of responsibility that override other valuable facets of social life. So whilst the transition from childhood to adulthood might be a discursive construction it has profound consequences for how we have fun—appropriate/inappropriate fun, the spaces for fun and inhibition/disinhibition are active in our views of how we either conform or transgress and how this then relates to fun.

Whilst the tenor was different between the stories from childhood and the stories from adulthood some of the central themes remain constant. 'Other people' and 'the outdoors' featured most frequently in both the adult and child fun, thus accentuating both the social and phenomenal sides of fun. It was interesting that family appeared less frequently in the adult data with friends becoming more important. As was mentioned in the previous chapter this is because familial adults are the arbiters of fun in childhood, and the family often provides the setting where fun happens. In adulthood the dependence on those people recedes as we become more responsible for creating the contexts within which fun happens ourselves. At the same time, with this increase in responsibility comes an awareness of age appropriateness and the rules of growing older. These twin processes serve to distance us from the fun of our childhoods and moves us into the more compartmentalised fun, the fun where flashes of disinhibition or transgressive behaviour are had knowingly and briefly. More often the fun described in adulthood was more sedentary than that in childhood. Talking and laughing featured but this again was a reflection of the fun of spending positive time with other people. There was more excitement conveyed in the narratives that involved holidays and trips, and as with childhood these were often with reference to specific others—family, partners and friends. There were elements that were clearly distinct from childhood. The role of alcohol, in many stories, points towards the need for assistance or an excuse when it comes to having disinhibited fun. This idea that it is difficult to shake off concerns or anxieties is a concern for many working in mental health, and the capacity to orient ourselves away from overanxiousness or a sense of too much responsibility is recognised as important. However, as the opportunities or capacity to have fun appear to be diminished in adulthood the consequences for us are clear.

The most prominent feature of the stories provided in the survey was the primacy of fun as a social activity. The narratives involved other people and the fun was inspired by, experienced with or directed towards others. The contexts within which the fun happens change, and circumstances are mediated through a variety of features of life—age, gender, class, and so on—but the core component of fun is that it is a social activity however that sociality is configured.

References

Aries, P. (1962). *Centuries of childhood: A social history of family life*. New York: Random House.

Becker, H. (1964). Personal change in adult life. *Sociometry, 27*(1), 40–53.

Bengtson, V., Elder, G., & Putney, N. (2012). The life course perspective of aging: Linked lives, timing and history. In J. Katz, S. Peace, & S. Spurr (Eds.), *Adult lives: A life course perspective*. Bristol: Policy Press.

Broner, M., & Tarone, E. (2001). Is it fun? Language play in a fifth-grade Spanish immersion classroom. *The Modern Language Journal, 85*(3), 363–379.

Elder, G. (1994). Time, human agency and social change: Perspectives on the life course. *Social Psychology Quarterly, 57*(1), 4–15.

Fincham, B., Langer, S., Scourfield, J., & Shiner, M. (2011). *Understanding suicide*. Basingstoke: Palgrave.

Johnson, M., Crosnoe, R., & Elder, G. (2011). Insights on adolescence from a life course perspective. *Journal of Research on Adolescence, 21*(1), 273–280.

Merleau-Ponty, M. (2002 [1945]). *Phenomenology of perception*. London: Routledge.

Neugarten, B., Moore, J, & Lowe, J. (1965). Age norms, age constraints, and adult socialization. *American Journal of Sociology, 70*(6), 710–717.

Office for National Statistics. (2013, July 30). Personal wellbeing in the UK, 2012-13. *ONS Statistical Bulletin*. http://www.ons.gov.uk/ons/dcp171778_319478.pdf. Accessed 12 Nov 2015.

Oesterle, S., Johnson, M, & Mortimer, J. (2004). Volunteerism during the transition to adulthood: A life course perspective. *Social Forces, 82*(3), 1123–1149

Wellard, I. (2013). *Sport, fun and enjoyment: An embodied approach*. London: Routledge.

5

Fun at Work

Work is not fun—they are not mutually inclusive concepts. Work is not intended to be fun. Definitions of work are notoriously slippery. As Strangleman and Warren suggest, it can mean effort or labour or more specifically what a person does to earn money (Strangleman and Warren 2008: 1). The ways in which we deploy the term are many and various. However, one thing that is not a definitional characteristic of work is fun. If a person does have fun whilst at work, this is a happy by-product of the real purpose of work—which is to be productive, in whatever form that might take. This is no more apparent than in the rhetoric of work/life balance. The term itself implies that work is a distraction from those other elements of life that are fulfilling, joyful and meaningful.

It is obvious that the mechanics and instruments of work and employment have changed over the decades. The disintegration of heavy industry in some parts of the world and its development elsewhere, the increasing reliance on information technologies and the disappearance of agrarian employment over the last century in Western Europe have at least altered the landscape of work. Despite this, there appear to be features of work that survive irrespective of changes in the nature of work. From glimpses into the past from literature and from data gathered for this project, fun and its unwelcome corollary boredom appear to be relatively resilient to change. Many observations on work from 60 or 70 years ago still resonate (Roy 1959; Baldamus 1961; Becker 1963; Illich 1975; Gorz 1999; Walker and Fincham 2011) with the affective responses to the debilitating effects of work and also distracted enjoyment at work unaltered in the face of the restructuring of forms of work that have developed in the same time frame. The rhetoric around our experiences of work have completed an about-face, so workplaces in Western Europe and North America increasingly concern themselves with creating happy or fun environments for people to work in. This is clearly different from the factory floors of previous eras, designed to be tolerable. Despite this partial volte-face, people are experiencing fun, at least in ways that clearly resonate with the past. How best to cope with 'the beast of monotony' (Roy 1959: 158) is a contemporary concern found not only in this study but also in the study that formed the basis for the book *Work and the Mental Health Crisis in the UK* (Walker and Fincham 2011). As was mentioned in the introduction, part of the impetus for thinking specifically about fun emerged during the study on mental health and work. In that study Carl Walker and I noticed that, at best, people felt ambivalent towards their jobs. At worst people hated them. However, there were persistent references made to moments in the day that either relieved boredom or made light of bad situations - in other words, moments of fun. In terms of trying to understand why it appeared to be uniformly experienced—rather than people mainly having fun at work punctuated by short bursts of boredom—Gi Baldamus provided an interesting perspective on the nature of our experiences of being at work. Rather than the normal state of affairs being one of cooperation and harmonious relationships, work is an environment structured by 'differentiated power that reflects unequally distributed advantages and disadvantages' (Baldamus 1961: 7). As Erickson succinctly notes from Baldamus:

> When we look in depth at what work actually involves for many, the meanings attached to work and the costs of work to the individual in terms of stress, workplace conflict, alienation and ill health, the real question we need to address isn't why people stop working, but why they work at all. (Erickson 2010: 36–7)

If we understand work from this perspective it becomes clear why our experiences of fun or levity in work are so fleeting. As Walker and I suggest:

> The resonance of this way of looking at work is clear. Rather than examining what is going wrong for people at work which would normally be characterised as positively functional, this perspective suggests examining what is good for people in an environment that is normally negatively functional. (Walker and Fincham 2011: 40–1)

In this characterisation of work there is no anticipation that the *experience* of work will be fulfilling or fun—irrespective of its symbolic construct[1]—in which case the generation of fun or punctuation of the day with moments of levity is exactly what ought to be expected. As will be illustrated, it is certainly the case that the people that were surveyed in this study understood fun as an infrequent moment of levity that broke the normal course of events.

Fun at Work in Context

There is a growing literature—largely American—on 'workplace fun'. The idea being that productivity might be increased by a concentration on creating an environment where the working day is punctuated by periods of 'fun'. This point of view has gained momentum as employers realise that it is a useful way of extracting more from people working for them. Since the 1980s there have been literally hundreds of management manuals demonstrating the benefits of providing fun at work. Amongst many, Weinstein provides a wonderful example of this literature in his 1997 book *Managing to Have Fun*. In this work he provides rationales and pointers for employees in the late 1990s informed largely in his participation with an organisation called Playfair:

---

[1] Work and employment are bound up with not only ideas of pay and task but also identity and self-respect/status. For the purposes of this argument I am talking about how we feel when we are at work rather than the more abstract or symbolic ideas that also surround work.

> I like to believe that the important questions businesspeople will ask in the next century will not just be about productivity, quality, or reengineering. I hope one of the questions will be 'Having fun?' because laughter and play and fun on the job can create a culture of caring and connection in the workplace that is just as important—if not more so—than productivity and profitability. 'Having fun?' is a powerful question, because it puts the primary value on the *people* in the organisation. It is a revolutionary question to be posed in the world of business. And once we begin to ask this question of ourselves as well as of each other then we can truly transform the way we live at work. (Weinstein 1997: 24)

Whilst this is an admirable sentiment, it is worth bearing in mind that the full title of the book is *Managing to have fun: How having fun at work can motivate you employees, inspire your co-workers, boost your bottom line*. The economic advantages of this managerial approach, whilst not foregrounded in the rhetoric, are always there. There are contrasts within this literature in the extent to which authors emphasise corporate instrumentalism, that is, fun at work is good for productivity, and corporate paternalism, that is, fun at work is good for the well-being of employees (Weinstein 1997; Newstrom 2002; Ford et al. 2003; Karl et al. 2005; Fluegge-Woolf 2014).

Whilst Google, Yahoo and Innocent may appear innovators with regard to providing recreational distractions for employees, this is far from a new phenomenon. Perhaps the most famous example of designing working environments to promote well-being, and associating it with productivity, is the development of Cadbury's Bournville site in the UK in 1879. As Cadbury's explain:

> Production began at the Cadbury Brothers' 'Bournville factory in a garden' in September 1879. When the workers arrived they found facilities that were simply unknown in Victorian times. There was a field next to the factory where men were encouraged to play cricket and football; a garden and playground for the girls; a kitchen where workers could heat up their meals, and properly heated dressing rooms where they could get changed. As George [Cadbury] said, 'If the country is a good place to live in, why not to work in?' (Cadbury.co.uk 2015)

The founders of Cadbury's, Richard and George Cadbury, actively promoted recreational and sporting activities to their employees providing facilities on site—however, the sporting pastimes were almost exclusively reserved for male employees. Over time men's and women's swimming pools were built, and alongside religious observance, the importance of health and what we might now call well-being was at the heart of Cadbury's commercial enterprise. As their website proudly trumpets, 'Cadbury duly became famous not just for its prosperity, but also for the advances in conditions and social benefits for its workforce' (Cadbury. co.uk.2015).

This philosophy—that employers have a responsibility for the well-being, and even happiness of workers, outside of the normal parameters of things like health and safety—has extended from Bournville's early experiments through companies such as Guinness and Hershey's in the twentieth century (Bolton and Houlihan 2009: 558) to a number of contemporary companies establishing working practices quite outside of the anticipated parameters of 'normal' working—and these philosophies have gone through three distinct phases. Bolton and Houlihan characterise the ethos of Cadbury's, Guinness and Hershey's as one of corporate paternalism where the role of social responsibility is the primary impetus for the implementation of working practices and environments that promote the well-being of employees. Through the 1970s and 1980s a corporate instrumentalism developed where firms like Hewlett-Packard initiated a more overt and event-based practice where the fun at work is more organised and designed specifically to maximise the productivity and ultimately profit of the corporation. More recently, and associated with the growing concern with work–life balance, a hybrid instrumentalism has developed, where the assumption is that the welfare of workers and the well-being of the corporation are more closely related. The more cynical deployment of fun at work in the 1980s has been largely replaced with a more amorphous discourse, where environments that promote the idea of a more autonomous form of fun-making are created. The extent to which this actually happens is contentious.

As I have said, Google, Yahoo and Innocent all promote ways of working that do not fit the stereotypical model of a clear and distinct line between working and enjoying oneself. In a book outlining Richard Branson's approach to employing people in his Virgin group John Dearlove says:

> Throughout his business life Richard Branson has managed to portray work as a social activity. Going to the office at Virgin isn't the drudgery that it can be at other companies, or at least, that's what Branson wants his people to believe and clearly believes himself. 'I get the best people, I ask questions, and then I say: "let's have some fun",' he explains. In the early days, low wages and run-down environments were compensated for by regular wild parties and a carnival atmosphere. Even today, the line between working life and social life is hard to draw at the company, Virgin staff work hard and play hard. (Dearlove 2002: 68)

In this passage Dearlove alerts us to an interesting facet of Branson's motivation for creating a fun environment to work in—to an extent it was to make up for poor working conditions. Wages were low and the places of work were run-down but the parties and the atmosphere compensated for these shortcomings. The role of productivity and what Andre Gorz calls subjection will be outlined later, but for all the philanthropic rhetoric provided by these sorts of employers the fun is not just for the benefit of the workers. There is a philosophy or perspective developing of how best to optimise human capital at work.

Interest in fun at work has grown in management literature as developments in the corporate sector have taken shape. Referred to variously as 'workplace', 'organised' or 'packaged' fun, this type of activity differs from the descriptions of fun that have been deployed here so far. It is clear that this managed, encouraged and monitored fun is distinct from what some have termed 'organic' fun (Bolton and Houlihan 2009; Stromberg and Karlsson 2009). For Bolton and Houlihan organic fun is already an intrinsic and inherent part of organisational life (Bolton and Houlihan 2009: 565) which already sets managed or organised fun apart from the thing that Walker and Guest referred to in 1952 on the assembly line in an automobile factory. There is spontaneity and control present when the workers said 'we have a lot of fun and talk all the time' (Walker and Guest 1952: 77) and 'if it weren't for the talking and fooling you'd go nuts' (Walker and Guest 1953: 68), and this stands in contrast to the sorts of 'organised' or 'packaged' fun that concerns Bolton and Houlihan. This is reflected in their contention that:

> Official fun has some striking features in the way it presumes that fun will be on managerial terms and that there will be benefits for all. (Bolton and Houlihan 2009: 565)

Sanctioned fun often needs tight policing lest it get out of control. There are boundaries of acceptability in the construction of organised fun. Plester quotes a manager at a law firm where the perception is that it is that they encourage people to have fun (Plester 2009: 588):

> We need to have a lot of young people and we need to have a lot of fun, but I still worry a bit when they get a little bit too loud and laughing too much that it is not quite professional and it might look perhaps that they are not doing much, to other people. (Plester 2009: 589)

For Plester a key issue in the manufacturing of fun for workers is that there is a line that can be crossed, and in a similar way that parents may scold their child, the employer will apply censure when they feel as though an employee has gone too far. This process feels antithetical to the ways in which we understand fun either in a common-sense way or the theoretical frame that was discussed in Chap. 2 of this book. The subversive and spontaneous is clearly absent from organised or packaged fun promoted by employers wishing to provide a particular atmosphere or culture within which productivity can thrive. There are tight cultural boundaries that are policed by institutional norms and expectations and these inhibit the sorts of fun that is celebrated by those having it. At the same time as the contrived organisation of fun in this context there is a belief that there is a causal relationship between happiness and productivity. This, whilst appearing sensible, is empirically unproven but a further assumption is that workplace fun will produce happy workers—thus improving productivity. Bolton and Houlihan question this assumption:

> As a result workplace engagement has transitioned from the classic realm of team nights out and sports and socials onto new terrain and raced forth with activities ranging from fancy dress days to 'Wacky Fridays', karaoke competitions, laughter workshops, exotic training events and encouragements to embrace our inner clown. (Bolton and Houlihan 2009: 557)

So the relationship between fun and workplaces touches on the issue of the management of fun contrasting with the idea of fun as spontaneous. It has also evolved through phases of managerial discourses of corporate responsibility, for example, the paternalism of Cadbury's, Guinness or Hershey's, to the corporate instrumentalism of the 1970s and 1980s, for example, Hewlett-Packard and 'beer busts', to a 1990s recession-inspired instrumentalism affirming a relationship between fun and productivity. The twenty-first-century manifestation of this relationship has relied on an influx of young, extremely successful entrepreneurs to create working environments where the infrastructure is supposed to encourage creativity through fun. Google, Ben and Jerry's and Innocent are examples of this phenomenon.

The advent of post-industrial working affords an opportunity for some employers to accentuate the social aspects of working. Famously, Google has created workspaces that look like play areas—incorporating features of play like slides and ping-pong tables as well as quirky interior designs and spaces to socialise and even sleep.

This trend for open plan, inventive and 'fun' working spaces has been replicated elsewhere. In the USA Twitter, Airbnb and Yahoo have constructed huge open plan working spaces filled with the apparatus of distraction—pool tables, swings, table tennis tables, slides, and so on. In the UK Innocent Drinks, Mind Candy and Red Bull, amongst others, have followed this model.

It is interesting to note that whilst these philosophies emerge sequentially, they do run concurrently. There are plenty of workplaces that deploy the sorts of 'fun' distractions of corporate instrumentalism (see Plester 2009). For some workplaces the relationship between fun and control is managed through the introduction of fun experts who come to workplaces and provide fun for employees. There are several companies offing such services. One 'Fun at Work Company' introduces its services to potential clients like this:

> *Put a smile on the face of all your staff.*
> Ideas from the weird and wacky, through to the active, competitive, cerebral and cultural. It's been well accepted that there is a direct relationship between 'fun at work' and employee motivation, productivity, creativity, satisfaction and retention. A planned programme of occasional and surprise activities at your workplace will bring staff, at all levels, to work with a *smile*, never knowing what might happen today. Humor is in the unexpected and it is well known to help relieve stress and improve health, there is little else that will make a person feel as good as a laugh. (Fun at Work Company 2015)

The motivation for employers to bring the Fun at Work Company is clear. The benefits are to be felt in areas of productivity. The explicit link between motivation, satisfaction and productivity once again brings to mind Gorz's thoughts on subjection in 'Reclaiming Work'—explained more fully later. In this scenario the worker feels an affiliation to the company that is treating them well and will try their hardest to maximise their productive capacity, thus benefitting the productive enterprise. However, as Gorz points out, this relationship is one way and exploitative. The concern for the welfare or happiness of the worker only lasts as long as it is economically or productively expedient to keep them happy. During changes in productive processes or economic climates the worker is an expendable resource and their welfare is no longer a concern of the productive enterprise. This is a reality that has been felt by many people who have suffered a stagnation of wages, less favourable conditions of employment or even job loss.

As I have suggested the empirical basis for the contention that fun is good for productivity is limited—and the for the sorts of events organised by people like the Fun at Work Company the scope for fun as has been earlier defined appears limited, to me at least. The role of fun at work—humour and game-playing—for many of us has a subversive element, and in the way that Donald Roy describes undermines managerial control (Roy 1959) rather than supports it as appears to be the case in organised or packaged fun. As Bolton and Houlihan suggest, fun is used to 'upset the status quo and to provide space for escape as much as a means for engagement' (Bolton and Houlihan 2009: 560). It should also be noted that the subjective experience of fun differs from person to person and whilst there may be joy and hilarity in organised workplace fun for some, it can 'create misery' for others (Bolton and Houlihan 2009: 560).

Work/Life Balance

Alongside the fun at work discourse, it is also thought that fun and happiness are (a) important for well-being and (b) within our grasp if we do the right thing. There is a prevailing discourse that there is a balance to be struck between the debilitating effects of work and overwork and home/rest of your life. In the study into mental health and work we asked a sample of workers about their work/life balance. Whilst they gave a variety of answers, the point here is that the term was meaningful to every one of them. There wasn't a single person that did not have an idea of what a work/life balance means (Walker and Fincham 2011). However, the increasing popularity of workplace fun or making the spaces or infrastructure of work fun suggests that there is a conceptual blurring of the neat distinction between work as bad for you and the rest of your life having to make up for this. With the advent of movements such as positive psychology, the deployment of fun as an incentive to increase productivity became fashionable:

> Research conducted into corporate culture in the early 1980s argued that the success of many blue chip US corporations was largely due to the intermix of work and play. As a result, the appropriate use of fun, play and humour came to be promoted in managerial literature as a resource that could be used positively to energise and motivate employees, increase employee well-being and contribute to economic performance. These strategies were adopted by a number of businesses in the US, the UK, and Australia. (Owler 2008: 40)

This is a distinctly different relationship to recreation than that of the corporate paternalism in Bournville and with several large and influential companies making explicit claims about the relationship between well-being, fun and profit. As has been mentioned, a number of corporations are at the forefront of promoting a very twenty-first-century interpretation of this—as is demonstrated by the growth in work spaces that are intended to blur the boundaries between work and play.

The benefits of working in environments that do not resemble workhouses or where employees feel as though the company has their best interests at heart are obvious. The ways in which well-being through fun are promoted relate not just to an oblique notion of well-being, but quite specific forms of identification. One is the forms of fun and what your engagement with them might say about you, but another is related to autonomy. Feeling as though an employer is sanctioning forms of activity away from tightly defined corporate or productive tasks generates feelings of autonomy away from identification with repetitive or soul-destroying meaningless or menial tasks. This does bring to mind the idea of traction as proposed by Gi Baldamus in *Efficiency and Effort* in 1961. In a similar vein to Erickson I think that Arlie Hochschild's thoughts on 'emotional labour' as defining some contemporary forms of labour is a very competent description of processes that have always been present since at least the development of industrial labour. The requirement of Hochschild's airline stewardesses to be happy and smiley for the customers is reminiscent of pretty much any service sector one cares to think of. An obvious example would be the required polite subservience of butlers and housemaids in Western Europe from the eighteenth century until the twentieth century. Whilst a different type of emotional management, it is emotional management as a requirement of the job nonetheless. In environments where there is a managed expectation of satisfaction, fun or happiness—this is a headline feature of the employment practice—it is important that the employees respond positively to initiatives. It is easy to be cynical about expectations to emotionally respond in positive ways in working environments, and assume that workers will not but Erickson cites studies where people are enjoying themselves at work. Whilst acknowledging the strengths of

Hochschild's work he suggests that there is more to explain than offered by emotional labour:

> The studies identify workers coping with their work environments, articulating their professional skills and interacting with a range of clients in different settings. And, perhaps most significantly, they have identified workers actually enjoying what they are doing. Perhaps what we are seeing is simply 'traction': people becoming caught up in their work and finding a mechanism, even a satisfaction to oppose the tedium they are experiencing. (Erickson 2010: 49)

At the centre of much of this thinking is the tacit assumption that work tasks are generally unfulfilling. So for Baldamus we create our own satisfaction through ideas of having done a good job, or having expertise in the mechanics of any given task. Rather than this being a distraction away from the productive task, this is a distraction into or towards the productive task. This sort of intrinsic distraction, away from associated feelings of disenfranchisement or boredom, is owned by the worker—it is their creative sensibility that enables traction to occur. This is distinct but related to the discourse of fun at work. In this there is also a tacit assumption that work tasks are unfulfilling but the distraction is obviously away from task. This is distinct again from gamification where attention is not distracted but focussed on the task transformed into a game[2] (Dale 2014).

The encouragement to have sanctioned fun at work involves the promotion of elements of life that are not inherently associated with work.

This does raise the question of why some employers feel it necessary or appropriate to provide facilities for distraction or fun, particularly if there are other ways of extracting efficient productivity. Despite there being a

---

[2] Gamification is a relatively new way of managing work that implies that productivity is enhanced by making everything a game. Whilst the merits of this approach are rehearsed elsewhere, the reason this book does not concentrate on it is that there is no suggestion of the imputation of fun in work that is not covered by the fun at work literature—the idea that productivity is increased if fun is instituted as a characteristic of work or workplaces.

distinct lack of empirical evidence supporting a direct causal link between fun and productivity there is a belief that there must be one. There is a particularly telling comment in a paper from a human resources journal where Ford, McLaughlin and Newstrom say this:

> An increasing body of evidence indicates a positive organisational environment of fun work culture is a valuable asset for organisations (Ford and Heaton). Luthans (2002) talks about the value of subjective well being (SWB) as a contributor to a positive organizational behaviour. The linkage between working in a fun work environment and having a sense of well being seems somewhat obvious and the SWB concept incorporates a number of factors such as life satisfaction, job satisfaction, and levels of experiencing pleasant emotions and moods (Diener). Other authors, like Perrin state that, 'Common sense supports the theory that having fun at work helps generate profitable business'. (Ford et al. 2003: 23)

Google's attitude to those working in their development units is well known, but they are committed to the idea that there *is* a causal link between happiness and productivity. In a report in the *New York Times* a spokesperson for Google was explicit about this:

> Google's various offices and campuses around the globe reflect the company's overarching philosophy, which is nothing less than 'to create the happiest, most productive workplace in the world', according to a Google spokesman, Jordan Newman. (*New York Times* 2013)

As has been mentioned, the discourse of fun at work, to be found in the many management philosophy literature, highlights a different sort of relationship to fun encouraged by employers and managers to employees (Weinstein 1997; Newstrom 2002; Ford et al. 2003; Karl et al. 2005; Fluegge-Woolf 2014). This is not the aggressive 'beer bust' culture of the 1980s, but a more joyful person-centred approach informed by concerns for work–life balance and both the physical and mental well-being of workers. Whilst this might be a reality in some cases, it is not how fun at work is being experienced more broadly. The discourse is useful in the sense that it can engender a sense of loyalty and being cared about. This is the process Andre Gorz calls subjection:

> In a disintegrating society, in which the quest for identity and the pursuit of social integration are continually being frustrated, the 'corporate culture' and 'corporate loyalty' inculcated by the firm offer the young workers a substitute for membership of the wider society, a refuge from the sense of insecurity. (Gorz 1999: 36)

Whilst the picture invoked by Gorz is more bleak than many would acknowledge, the idea that our loyalty is to an extent bought by our employers is perhaps more easy to agree with. In accord with Dearlove's inadvertent suggestion that people want to work for Richard Branson because he provided things that other employers did not—except for good wages and conditions (Dearlove 2002: 68), Gorz suggests that as traditional bonds between people loosen there is space for new configurations and this gap is being filled by loyalty to a hierarchical structure, the corporation—which is not at its core loyal to the worker. Of interest to this book are the ramifications for individuals' experiences of work in the face of subjection. For Gorz the worker must demonstrate loyalty or face the consequences, but increasingly a demonstration of loyalty is an adoption of particular identities that chime with the overall corporate identity. When it comes to fun the demonstration that you know when to have fun and how to have fun is important for knowing whether you fit or not. The 'freedom' apparently afforded to workers at Google, for example, to have fun is not how most workers in the UK at least experience fun at work. As will be illustrated later in the chapter, the sorts of fun described here is even more muted than the change in tone from the stories in childhood to the stories in adulthood. Occasional events or dressing up days, teambuilding days or counterpoised with the actual fun—mucking about, having a break, not doing what you are supposed to. The relationship between subjection, appropriate fun having and Wolfenstein's fun morality is clear. There is a tacit policing of fun at work where the demonstration of identity and a particular orientation to fun is determined by a corporate culture that does not bear any relation to freedom, autonomy, transgression or naughtiness—sometimes it masquerades as the same thing. In a particularly gruesome episode of a BBC 'fly-on-the-wall' documentary *The Call Centre*, the manager of a large call centre in South Wales, Nev, explains that he gets all new employees to stand in a room together and sing a pop song—this event is shown in the episode. When explaining what this has to do with working in a call centre, Nev says:

> Each new recruit has to sing, I don't even care if they're in the admin jobs, it's a fact, they've got to sing. Each new recruit sings and I want enthusiasm. Enthusiastic people sell, happy people sell, miserable bastards can't. If they can't sing and they can't enjoy it they might as well leave. (BBC 3—*The Call Centre* 2013)

He then goes on to explain how he sacked two women from their call centre jobs for not singing. In conversation with young people about their experiences of trying to get jobs it turns out that this sort of practice is not uncommon. Notable examples being a young woman having to make up and perform a rap to get a temporary job in a catering outlet and a man and a woman independently telling me that they had to perform jokes to a number of potential managers in the hope of getting a job in a chain pub/bar.

As will be illustrated, most people do not work in places that provide facilities for distraction or fun—in the way that Google, Yahoo, Innocent or Red Bull claim to, but many employers are aware that there is something in fun, or at least in enjoyable distraction, that requires some lip service paid. It is not uncommon in the UK to find large employers allowing workers to dress up or have organised fun either for morale or for charity.

Experiences from My Data

As part of the survey I conducted about fun, I asked people about fun whilst at work. As has been mentioned, the sample of 201 came from a range of occupational backgrounds and covered a range of ages. The ways in which people described having fun at work fell into six broad categories: banter, subversion, discrete activities, play, time away and don't have fun. It was interesting that the variation in reported experiences was not nearly as wide as I had anticipated—that may have something to do with way the question was phrased—but also might have something to do with the persistence of uniformity in working practices and therefore uniformity in resisting Baldamus' 'tedium'. As is often the case with qualitative analysis, there is much overlap between the discrete categories that I have used to describe the data—this has been a particular issue for this project, where definitions of fun deployed by respondents to the survey themselves have been fluid.

Talking/Chatting/Banter/Joking

A high proportion of respondents to the question 'If you work, how do you have fun at work?' identified verbal actions as being the primary locus of their fun at work. This included 'talking', 'chatting', 'banter' and 'joking'. This reported form of fun was the most prevalent in the cohort (47/201). There was a distinction in the ways in which people deployed the terms banter on the one hand and chatting or talking on the other.

It might seem reasonable to assume that chatting and talking are the same, and there is clearly huge overlap between how these two terms are deployed; however, there are subtle differences in the data between the two. For a start some people referred to both in their statements as though they were different or as if referring to chatting augmented the nature of the talk. Talking was less playful. Some referred to clients or customers, 'by talking to customers and colleagues about what they're buying or what they're up to' (F20, Student and shop assistant). These examples are typical of the non-distractive deployment of talk as fun. However, another person mentioned talking as distinct from laughing and joking, 'talking to colleagues, laughing and joking—being close. The last few years have been so troubled that this is probably support and survival at the moment rather than fun' (F49, Academic). Given that this person has experienced difficulties at work, the distinct phenomenon of talking, laughing and joking are important as co-constitutive elements of support.

It is the case that when people mentioned 'talking' they referred to work tasks, customers or colleagues. The focus of the 'talk' was not necessarily away from tasks associated with work. More than talking, chatting was associated with distraction or time away from focussed, work-oriented tasks. Chats, or talking, over lunch or break times was mentioned by several respondents; one said in response to the question 'how do you have fun at work?' 'having a coffee with colleagues, chatting in the corridor, basically when I meet people I like talking to (F30, Researcher). Another said, 'general chit chat can be fun sometimes. Sometimes staff days out, depending on what we do' (F48, Administrator).

Most of the respondents that mentioned chatting did not ascribe any other purpose to it than enjoyment or distraction. A few did, however, intimate that this form of fun served other purposes. A researcher said 'chats over coffee break, sharing experiences with colleagues. Laughing off problems that emerge' (F29, Researcher). In this instance the chatting is important for getting a sense of perspective on issues arising at work, and talking through problems in a light-hearted way. Another suggested there was further utility in chatting, outside of simple distraction with the idea of networking. In response to the question:

> Chatting to workmates, going for walks and seeing people to have a chat to. Meeting friends for lunch. I call it networking, others call it gossip and chat. (F33, Facilities co-ordinator)

As with all of the other forms of fun as defined by respondents there was often a sense that fun happened despite work—a fairly traditional view of work and fun as incommensurate:

> It's not so fun these days. Lots of time pressures and worried people. Else chatting gossiping. (F43, Lecturer)

As has been mentioned before, the interactional element to fun is large—it almost always requires other people. The number of times that talking and chatting were mentioned is interesting for a couple of reasons. The first is that it is not something that people reported as fun when they were asked to describe fun—it only occurs when people are asked to think about work. Chatting does not require physicality; it can occur in quite restrictive settings and, I have to say, is a pretty poor substitute for the sorts of things that were reported elsewhere in the survey.

One person highlighted the contextual nature of experiences inside and outside of work as being qualitatively different:

> Not much, no. From time to time I laugh or feel happy but I wouldn't categorise it the same way as having fun outside of work. (M44, Lecturer)

Whilst there is something very benign about descriptions of chatting and talking, those describing banter as a means of fun at work appeared much more active in their generation or pursuit of fun. One respondent described 'hilarious banter' (M35, IT manager) and others talked of conditions that create the conditions for banter. One said:

> Banter with colleagues, pretend arguments, pretending that the [boss] is on the phone, fantasy football rivalries and stupid e-mails. (M49, Lecturer)

Another accentuated the humorous element to banter:

> Joking with people, a lot of spoken human about all sorts of stuff [sic]. I would say that's most of it. There are aspects of my job that I think 'ooh this is really good' a satisfying task, completion. But I don't think of that as 'fun', fun is more interaction—piss-taking, dry humour, banter with colleagues. (M54, IT engineer)

Whilst another suggested that he actively created conditions for fun and banter:

> I have fun through conducting breaches [sic], banter with co-workers under pressure. (M32, student)

Whilst banter carries more playful and subversive connotations than mere chatting, it was most often used as a foil to expressing a paucity of fun at work. This was clearly expressed by many of the respondents to the survey, where banter was presented as the sole expression of fun:

> Rarely. I find work interesting but I wouldn't describe it as fun. I sometimes have fun when having 'banter' with colleagues, though the topic of our conversation is often work related. (M30, economist)

There is a sense of resignation in many of the less enthusiastic reports from the survey:

> I don't really! There is sometimes a bit of 'banter' at work but I wouldn't say that there was ever much 'fun' in the actual workplace, and only limited fun in work social events.

The response below was typical of the kind of short answers to the question of fun at work, with slightly deflated attitude being expressed by a number of respondents:

> Beyond corridor banter, not much (M46, University lecturer)

A surprising aspect of this thread of responses is, first, the lack of diversity in these people's experiences of fun at work when they report talk as the primary locus of their fun—there is uniformity to the ways in which talking, chatting and banter are described—second, when several people identified banter as how they had fun it was set against the idea that generally they did not have fun at work. So banter is not enough for people to imagine that they have fun whilst they are at work. As is illustrated, this was not universally the case, but enough people expressed this view for it to be of note.

Humour

Humour was frequently mentioned as being an important method for workers to have fun, but often in relation to chatting and gossiping. A key component of humour as a locus for fun-making is that it does not need much level of organisation, unlike games, play or fun-making involving elaborate props. Many people mentioned the term 'having a laugh' with others in answer to the question 'how do you have fun at work?', whilst other people described how humour played a role in their having fun at work. One public sector employee said 'humour or colleagues. Taking the piss out of myself' (M43, Social worker), whilst another person said 'playing pranks on other coworkers or sending around joke emails'

(F28, Graphic designer). It is obvious that, as with the other forms of fun expressed here, relationships with other people are essential, as one worker in Higher Education rather sadly said, 'Hmmmm....messing about with colleagues? I think relationships have to be established first, not there yet' (F35. Lecturer).

Subversion/Naughty/Undermining Boss or Rules

The richest source of narratives in relation to work and fun were those that highlighted the more subversive nature of having fun. These excerpts tended to focus on examples of events or practices to convey how fun was experienced. An important element for some was undermining authority, best represented by their bosses. One person said 'gossip with colleagues, make fun of management etc., go out for drinks' (F30, Academic), whilst another suggested that work is normally experienced in negative terms, but that camaraderie against authority in part compensated saying 'work is for most people dull and crap, myself included, but luckily the people make it good, and ganging up on the boss is always "fun"' (O25, Shop assistant). Whilst others highlighted the freedom afforded to workers when they are not being closely monitored, one said:

> Fun at work as a specific activity tends to be snuck in as small chunks e.g. a funny conversation when a manager is not there or a post it note wall of funny comments. There are lots of jokes and general teasing as we are all quite close. (F27, Schools outreach worker)

Another also suggested that fun happened outside of the managerial gaze and also mentioned another theme that frequently occurred, customers and/or clients:

> 'When the cat's away the mice will play', we dance to the store music when no customers are here, we joke about the nutty customers, we use the products on each other. (4 female, 20, Shop assistant)

Yet another highlighted the change in atmosphere when the boss was not present:

> Because I do different types of unpaid work, I shall only mention the work where I have fun, there is a lot that I do which is not fun. But working at Vinnies can be fun if the boss is not there, we try on clothes, joke with customers and enjoy ourselves. (45 Female, 71, Retired schoolteacher)

The capacity to be playful or behave outside of the normal strictures of the client/service provider relationship appears to be important for many working in such sectors. There were some that alluded to mocking customers. One said, 'I have fun at work by not taking things too seriously and I use sarcasm to have a laugh with the other waitresses,' whilst others were more explicit: 'Laughing—taking the p**s out of difficult clients, having lunch/drinks together' (F44, Architect). One waitress mentioned game playing as well as customers:

> My work is generally quite a fun atmosphere anyway but to have fun we might have small competitions to add a competitive aspect to the day. This doesn't always work, you have to be in the right mood and to get engaged otherwise it's not very fun. Also there is a transgressive element to the fun that I have at work for example talking when we are not supposed to or being inappropriate with customers. (F22, Student and waitress)

This person identified that transgression is an important part of experiencing fun in this context. It is interesting that she is aware that, with her colleagues, the fun is derived through crossing the boundary from appropriate to inappropriate to the expectations of the relationship with the customer. It is a question of power in this context. Along with the architect previously, the subservient role necessarily adopted in the customer–service provider context these people are challenging the power dynamic, albeit without the knowledge of the customer, and resting some control over their experience of the relationship through transgressive fun. Another respondent talked about their work in pubs:

> I've worked in pubs for years, and the best thing about it is having fun with my colleagues. We often stay drinking after work when the shift is finished,

and many of my close friends I've met through work. Because of the nature of the type of emotional labour involved with working in the service industry, often a lot of fun is gained from feeling like a team, in compared with the clientele [sic], who can often be rude, or drunk. Knowing there's people who understand and can joke about someone's rudeness, it makes something at times straining into a lot of fun. (F24, Barstaff)

In this excerpt the mention of emotional labour draws attention to the types of subversion that are available to such workers. The social aspect of work is particularly important in these contexts; it is in teams or with co-workers that empathy is developed and then a knowing humour or subversive activity emerges as a sort of coping strategy. This seems to me very similar to the observation of Walker and Guest about the production line—'if it weren't for the talking and fooling you'd go nuts'. The fun, in whatever form it takes, provides a platform for relief from the tedium or 'dull and crap' jobs (O25, Shop assistant) that many people have.

Colleagues and co-workers were also the objects of this more active fun-making process. There is an element of cruelty in the accounts of situations where other workers' discomfort is the source of fun for others. A supermarket worker said:

I work on the checkouts at Sainsburys, and find it quite fun winding up colleagues known as 'runners' (the people not serving on a checkout, but who hang around and swap items for customers who are at the checkout). Sending them on pointless errands can be fun. (F21, Student and part-time supermarket checkout worker)

Another person suggested that there was some equalising out or turn taking in the schadenfreude of their workplace, saying 'normally we "rib" someone, it depends on the day as to whose turn it is. Everyone is on the receiving end at some point in the week!' (F41, Vocational learning manager). A woman that worked part-time in kitchens said, 'Talking to the people I work with, being a bit mischievous and playing practical jokes in the kitchen' (F19, Student).

An account from an assistant in a shoe shop makes for excellent reading. In this account she encapsulates much of the tone and experiences of the sorts of subversive behaviour that make some forms of work more bearable:

> I work part time in a shoe shop. I have listed some of the things I do to have fun at work: 1) When we use the walkie-talkies, we tell jokes etc. that the customers can't hear. For example, yesterday my colleague started making creepy noises down the walkie, and no one could work out who it was. And one week, everyone saying chat-up lines that were related to shoes e.g. 'Hey Millie, your laces untied? Let me tie those for you, because I don't want to hear you falling for anyone else'. Everyone who has a walkie on can hear these things, and they all start laughing. 2) When we're in the stock room, we hide behind the racks and scare each other. 3) In the stock room, we push boxes off the shelves and onto each other's heads. 4) New stock arrives in massive boxes, and sometimes people hide in them and jump out on other unexpected workers [sic]. 5) If a good song comes on, we sometimes dance on the shop floor when customers have their backs turned. 6) People who work upstairs in the stock room send us funny messages down the shoe chute, and we send messages back up to them in the lift. (F21, Student and part-time sales assistant)

In terms of preconceived notions of ideal responses to this small survey I anticipated accounts that accentuated subversion or undermined authority would be more prevalent. As I have shown, they are here, but I had thought that practically all of the accounts would be full of these stories of naughtiness and mischief. However, only about a quarter of respondents reported this sort of proactive fun-making. It is clear that, for the people quoted above, challenging power or authority—bosses, clients or customers—is important and represented an important part of their experience of work as fun. It certainly stands in contrast to the organised or packaged fun promoted in much of the managerial literature of the last 20 years.

Play/Games

Related to mischief-making is game-playing. Whilst not subversive necessarily, there is a productive element to game-playing. It also appeals to the idea of childishness as being the lynchpin of having fun.

This is, of course, not an accurate account of having fun or playing games—adults have always thrived in play, just as children have. In fact several respondents worked with children and associated the game-playing with the children as part of their experience of fun at work. These accounts ranged from very short statements—as though playing with children and fun are self-evident, 'At work, play with children' (F34, Teacher at Child Care Centre) to longer accounts that outlined the infrastructure that supports the fun-making:

> I babysit so almost all I do is have fun. I get to play with new, cool toys and to teach someone younger than me how to use them. I read bed-time stories that [are] even more fun when you're a bit grown up. (F20, Student and child minder)

Most people do not work in environments where playing games are part of the job. Many people invent games using mundane tasks that make up their jobs. These accounts tended to be dominated by people working in education settings, both schools and Further Education/Higher Education settings. A teacher simply said that she had fun at work by 'being silly' (F39, Schoolteacher), whilst a student and part-time worker suggested that with others she spent time 'turning boring seeming activities into games, such as playing buzzword bingo or similar' (F40, Student). Another said 'making up games with co-workers; playing sports etc.' (M30, Lecturer). A schoolteacher said 'joking around with colleagues; playing games with language when teaching or learning; or simply playing games' (M40, Schoolteacher). The games that people played ranged from language play to more elaborate and physical games. One respondent explained, 'We had a game of "office olympics" at my suggestion last weekend. Myself and another [person], diving onto swivel chairs. I got carpet burn' (F31, Teacher and PhD student).

They also involved machines normally used for productive tasks:

> I work full time and I love my job. Fun can be simple pleasures like seeing a new flower or an insect. I never go anywhere without my camera, and later I post my photos on Flickr and enjoy the responses of viewers. Fun can also be the interaction with customers. And fun can be driving

the forklift or having silly races, riding the trolleys! Or it might be sharing a silly moment with my colleagues. (F59, Plant area manager in a garden centre)

The game-playing described here is a consistent feature of people creating entertaining distractions from their tasks at work throughout the era of industrial labour, and it was in organised games that the paternalistic employees—such as Guinness and Cadbury's—saw an outlet for frustrations that workers may have felt in the routinised industrial labour process. However, even when distractions are sanctioned, workers still invent their own ways of making boring tasks interesting or taking themselves away from tasks demanded by either employers or the work itself.

Breaks/Time Away from Productive Activities

Another area that was frequently mentioned were the times away from work tasks, such as lunchtime or other sanctioned breaks in the working day. Several respondents answered the question 'how do you have fun at work?' by simply answering 'lunch break' or 'coffee time'. The associated social interaction was mentioned, 'coffee time! Good coffee, biscuits and catch up with all the gossip' (F45, Senior research officer), others mentioned time away from colleagues, one admin worker said, 'I browse the internet when in the office and I take myself off for a walk in the park/woods if I have the time' (F36, Administrative assistant). Apart from the mention of social drinking after work, highlighted by three respondents, only one person talked about an organised activity during a sanctioned break: 'Very occasionally we play football during a lunchtime' (M41, IT technician).

There was a large crossover between those that reported sanctioned breaks and those that accentuated the role of gossiping or chatting as being important to their experience of fun—and the division between the two is indistinct in this analysis. However, there were enough people (15) that only wrote the break in the working day without explaining what happened in that time to warrant the identification of separate sections—breaks and chatting.

Discrete Activities or Occurrences/ Goal Orientation?

The relatively frequently cited source of fun at work was from positive orientation to work or work tasks. There were many mentions of satisfaction with a job well done, or that the job itself was fun. As an engineer pointed out, 'I generally have fun because I chose a profession whose main task is what I enjoy' (M57, Engineer) and an artist said 'talking to co-workers that you enjoy, enjoying what you're working on' (F28. Crafter/artist).

A number of respondents identified meeting objectives in work as fun, and for some this was associated with a level of self-direction. One person said they had fun 'by completing tasks I set for myself' (M26, Mature student) and a writer said, 'Writing, my work, is also the best fun. When it is flowing, the adrenalin gets going and time passes in a flash' (F66, Writer). An ICT consultant also highlighted the importance of control in making aspect of work fun; he had fun 'in conversation with friends and in steering projects towards topics and clients with whom I share an interest' (M55, ICT consultant). In all three of these examples there is a level of control or autonomy being indicative of a positive orientation to particular tasks or jobs. This is a well-documented source of satisfaction for workers. Gorz gives a good account of this process in the Volvo Uddavella plant experiment (Gorz 1999), and it is also an element of experiences of work that has been widely acknowledged in recent managerial literature (Landeweerd and Boumans 1994; Pearson and Moomaw 2005; Vidal 2013; Wu et al. 2015). Given this interest and the raft of recommendations that flow from this literature it is surprising that it did not feature more heavily as people's response to the question 'how do you have fun at work?'

A couple of people equated fun with some form of accomplishment or success; a police officer said, 'Doing as best as I can at work. Feeling accomplished' (M35, Police officer), whilst a physical therapist said:

> Fun at work is probably equated with some success. Either personal or patient related i.e. a patient achieves a goal! I might say 'that was fun'. Teaching is fun when I see the students interact and work together to

achieve a goal or crack a problem. Fun at work means time goes fast. (F48, Physical therapist)

A writer suggested that she had fun 'meeting new people, learning, overcoming challenges, winning battles' (F46, Freelance writer and carer). A striking feature of these sorts of contributions is that the problem-solving and success at work as fun are to do with other people's problems. There is not a concentration on the workers' own issues, rather a solving or successful resolution to somebody else's. In terms of the schema of fun described in Chap. 2 this involves a temporary alleviation from commitment and responsibility from personal anxieties or concerns.

There were two people that mentioned singing as part of their fun at work; one talked about directing a gospel choir organised through their work (F49, Senior technical officer) and a community arts worker said:

> I stand in the middle of a large circle of people. I make them laugh and I teach them beautiful harmonies. Instant positive feedback, and active participation are fun parts of my work. (F38, Community arts worker)

This last quote draws attention to the importance of fairly instant gratification in experiencing work as fun. Fun is experienced in the moment—that might be the moment of traction experienced by the writer when her work is 'flowing' or the teacher when they can see a problem solved by students. As is discussed on the chapter on theorising fun, the temporal nature of the distinctions between fun, happiness and pleasure are important for making sense of these accounts, but it is equally important to recognise that respondents themselves had difficulty in drawing those distinctions themselves. On the survey the order of questions meant that respondents answered questions of experiences before they were asked about definitions and distinctions. It could be the case that some people would have given more involved answers if they had been asked to unpick their experiences as fun, happy and/or pleasurable earlier. That said, the answers that they provided have given a valuable insight into how people are experiencing work outside of the anticipation of their experiences as mediated through managerial strategies or business rationales. Two of the most striking things about the accounts are, first, how traditional and conservative they seem. There is not an overwhelming sense of some sort of paradigm shift in the ways people are experiencing work as distinct from earlier periods. Second is the underwhelming nature of many of the accounts—work on the whole does not sound like much fun.

Don't Have Fun

In terms of a uniform response, 'I don't' was the most heavily used. A caveat to reading too much into this response is that, given that this was a self-complete, open-ended questionnaire, I did not have the opportunity to follow up on these responses. I suspect that if pushed, most people would have been able to identify elements of their working life that were fun; like Baldamus, I think that most people will create their own sense of satisfaction or amusement irrespective of the corporate objectives of employers. However, it is telling that a large proportion of the respondents to this questionnaire (20% of those that answered the question) answered that they did not have fun at work. Examples range from a student advisor who said 'I can't remember the last time I had fun at work. Socialising with colleagues OUTSIDE of work is fun though' (F49, Student advisor at an FE college) to the social worker who said 'I don't have fun at work, we have fun after work with colleagues sometimes' (F40, Social worker). Again, for a proofreader, fun was located outside of work, 'I don't really! There is sometimes a bit of "banter" at work (both roles) but I wouldn't say that there was ever much "fun" in the actual workplace, and only limited to social events' (M26, Property company proofreader). Similarly, an administrator highlighted that fun happened with colleagues, but outside of work: 'I wouldn't really have fun at work per se but I guess it's nice to just try to have a laugh with colleagues' (F40, Administrator). For some there was a sense that things had got worse over time; a lecturer said, 'It's not so fun these days. Lots of time pressures and worried people. Else chatting gossiping' (F43, Lecturer). There was an interesting perspective offered by a psychologist where she felt as though her professional status would be compromised if she were seen to be having fun. She said:

I don't have 'fun' at work as I think this would be at odds with acting in a professional way. I think having fun means doing something you don't expect and being free and disinhibited to experience that in any way that arises. I don't think this fits with being at work. (F41, Clinical psychologist)

There were several people that expressed the lack of fun in their work in fairly blunt terms. A shop assistant said in response to the question 'how do you have fun at work?', 'Saying to myself: I am not here, this isn't happening,' (F19, Shop assistant) and another said, 'By leaving'.

Conclusion

As might be expected, many of the themes presented here echo themes that emerged in the adult fun data, but they were mediated by the institutional expectations of work. Banter and chatting were almost inextricably linked to break times or times away from work. Fun talk happens in moments sanctioned by schedules of work or as an act of transgression or subversion. Nobody gave any hint that free talking or chatting was something that could happen or was encouraged in work time. So, the relationship between fun and subversion was, as might be expected, much more pronounced in the work data than in the fun in adulthood data. This is not surprising, as the fun in adulthood question did not imply that the generation of fun was necessarily inhibited by anything or anyone else—this is clearly the case in fun at work. The requirement to be productive inhibits, restricts or directs fun. Subversion then is a much stronger theme in these data than in any of the other data gathered in this project. Whilst I was amused by the stories, it is also sad to think that it is still the case that it is in opposition to authority that we can find fun—to me that does not say an awful lot for the evolution of management if the relationship that people have to work is the same as it was in the 1950s, even if forms of work have changed drastically.

Related to subversion was playing and games. It was often the case that games were invented and played in clear contravention of expected working norms. Messing about on furniture or mocking customers is as much subversive as it is creative—and is clearly a distraction strategy. Looming large overall of this data is Roy's 'Beast of Monotony', and our response to it appears, at least in this data, to be relatively uniform. The variety of ways in which fun was derived diminished in the data from considerations in childhood to considerations in adulthood to considerations of fun at work.

Much of the content in these data has to do with time away from productive tasks—however fleeting those times might be. It is interesting that many people that work at computers these days are astonished at their capacity for browsing web pages that have nothing to do with their jobs. I have had several conversations with people who complain that the BBC News website does not update quickly enough—because they find themselves reading the same thing so many times a day—rather than getting on with the productive task at hand.

It is worth reflecting on the model of fun presented in Chap. 2, *Theorising Fun*. The ways in which the data on fun at work fit with this model are striking.

In terms of a relationship to interaction, whilst less people were referred to directly in the data, the activities and moments that were listed almost certainly involved others. It is unlikely that when a respondent mentioned banter at break times they meant banter by themselves and to themselves. Similarly, the subversion or naughtiness that was mentioned was almost always for the benefit of joint fun—mockery or distraction. Time is a large factor in these data. The snippets of time eked out either away from the gaze of a boss or in a sanctioned break defined the space for fun. In fact, if time was not so heavily sanctioned or policed, the subversion of not doing what you are supposed to, when you are supposed to, would not be so appealing. The relative lack of free time makes both the free time valuable for having a particular type of sanctioned fun and productive time valuable for a particular type of subversive or transgressive fun.

As work is heavily repetitive, even in jobs that are characterised as varied, deviation from the norm is important, but quite complex. For many people the fun itself is repeated time and again. Much like 'in jokes' the observation by Blythe and Hassenzahl that fun is repetitive and non-progressive is important for understanding its relationship to norms.

So it is not that deviation from the norm means deviation from anything that one normally does, but deviation from the expected norm or value. In the case of this chapter the norm is that you buckle down and do your job, and the deviation from it is the fun that you and a colleague have every time you work a shift together.

In terms of commitment to productive tasks the fun described here always involves a temporary alleviation from that commitment. It is a knowing suspension of a commitment to task, which will end when we either choose to or are made to refocus. Associated to commitment is the idea of responsibility—and this is manifest in present concerns or anxieties. In relation to work, these concerns can be large or trivial—the scale of them is not important, the temporary alleviation of concentration on these concerns is. In the space created by this distraction, we have fun. This fun is manifest again away from the productive task. So the anxiety or concern can be, on the one hand, how to manage boredom, and on the other hand, how to solve a difficult problem—either way, fun operates as the tool for distraction away from these concerns.

The anticipation of fun at work tends to have a fairly formulaic quality. When we have fun outside of institutional settings the anticipation of what possibilities there are for situations or actions are far greater than when we are in institutional settings. It appears as though the capacity for creativity, let alone the opportunity for creativity, is stifled. In that respect anticipation takes on a more assuredly predictive flavour. We know that break time is coming, we know that a couple of our friends will be there and we know that we expect that we will talk and laugh—and frankly, for many of the respondents to my survey that was as good as it got.

Unlike fun in adulthood more generally, and to a certain extent fun in childhood, the sort of fun people had at work appeared less to do with choice and, as a consequence, identity and more to do with limited opportunities. That said, the idea that being known as a 'fun person' is mediated in very different ways, for example, between genders at work, suggests that it is still very important. However, this is less related to what a person does for fun or experiences fun, and more about how they are perceived as being fun.

This is the most obvious feature of the schema of fun that is represented in the data, and more obliquely in literature. Fun provides the backdrop for the distraction required for many people to keep going during the day in jobs that are not much fun otherwise.

Comparing literature on creating fun workplaces and then what people say about their experiences of fun at work illustrates a disconnect between the two. The fun that employers promote or facilitate and the fun that people actually have are two different things. The organised fun encouraged in management consultancy literature and the creative, subversive, distracted fun of employees are related in word alone. The objectives, generation and experience of each are distinct.

The unhappy conclusion of this chapter is that work does not appear to be that much fun for people today in pretty much the same way that it hasn't been for generations of workers before us.

References

Baldamus, W. (1961). *Efficiency and effort: An analysis of industrial administration*. London: Tavistock Publications.
BBC3. (2013). 'The Call Centre' on Youtube Happy People Sell—The Call Centre Episode One BBC 3, https://www.youtube.com/watch?v=6giqmaLzS50. (uploaded 4th June 2013) Accessed 9 Feb 2015.
Becker, H. (1963). *Outsiders*. New York: Free Press.
Bolton, S., & Houlihan, M. (2009). Are we having fun yet? A consideration of workplace fun and engagement. *Employee Relations, 31*(6), 556–568.
Cadbury.co.uk. (2015). Cadbury: The story. Available at https://www.cadbury.co.uk/the-story. Accessed 12 Jan 2015.
Dale, S. (2014). Gamification: Making fun work or making fun of work? *Business Information Review, 31*(2), 82–90.
Dearlove, D. (2002). *Business the Richard Branson way*. Chichester: Capstone.
Erickson, M. (2010). Efficiency and effort revisited. In M. Erickson & C. Turner (Eds.), *The sociology of Wilhelm Baldamus*. Farnham: Ashgate.
Fluegge-Woolf, E. (2014). Play hard, work hard: Fun at work and job performance. *Management Research Review, 37*(8), 683–705.
Ford, R., Mclaughlin, F., & Newstrom, J. (2003). Questions and answers about fun at work. *Human Resource Management*. Available at http://homepages.se.edu/cvonbergen/files/2012/12/Questions-and-Answers-about-Fun-at-Work1.pdf. Accessed 02 Nov 2015.

Fun at Work Company. (2015). Are you getting enough? http://www.funatwork.co.uk. Accessed 21 Jan 2015.

Gorz, A. (1999). *Reclaiming work: Beyond the wage based society*. Cambridge: Polity Press.

Illich, I. (1971). *Deschooling society*. Harmondsworth: Penguin.

Illich, I. (1975). *Tools for Conviviality*. London: Fontana.

Landeweerd, J., & Boumans, N. (1994). The effect of work dimensions and need for autonomy on nurses' work satisfaction and health. *Journal of Organizational and Occupational Psychology, 67*, 207–217.

Karl, K., Peluchette, J., Hall, L., & Harland, L. (2005). Attitudes towards workplace fun: A three sector comparison. *Journal of Leadership and Organizational Studies, 12*(2), 1–17.

New York Times. (2013). Looking for a lesson in Google's perks. *New York Times Online* http://www.nytimes.com/2013/03/16/business/at-google-a-place-to-work-and-play.html?_r=0. Accessed 01 Nov 2015.

Newstrom, J. (2002). Making work fun: An important role for managers. *The Society for the Advancement of Management Journal, 67*(1), 4–8.

Owler, K. (2008, April). Fun at work. *New Zealand Management* (p. 40–2).

Pearson, L. C., & Moomaw, W. (2005). The relationship between teacher autonomy and stress, work satisfaction, empowerment and professionalism. *Educational Research Quarterly, 29*(1), 37–53.

Plester, B. (2009). Crossing the line: Boundaries of workplace humour and fun. *Employee Relations, 31*(6), 584–599.

Roy, D. (1959). "Banana time": Job satisfaction and informal interaction. *Human Organization, 18*, 158–168.

Strangleman, T., & Warren, T. (2008). *Work and society: Sociological approaches, themes and methods*. London: Routledge.

Strömberg, S., & Karlsson, J. C. (2009). Rituals of fun and mischief: the case of the Swedish meatpackers. *Employee Relations, 31*, 632–647.

Vidal, M. (2013). Low-autonomy work and bad jobs in postfordist capitalism. *Human Relations, 66*(4), 587–612.

Walker, C., & Fincham, B. (2011). *Work and the mental health crisis in Britain*. Oxford: Wiley Blackwell.

Walker, C. R., & Guest, R. H. (1952). *The man on the assembly line*. Cambridge: Harvard University Press.

Weinstein, M. (1997). *Managing to have fun*. New York: Fireside.

Wu, C.-H., Griffin, M., & Parker, S. (2015). Developing agency through good work: Longitudinal effects of job autonomy and skill utilization on locus of control. *Journal of Vocational Behaviour, 89*, 102–108.

6

Phenomenal Fun

Whilst the social manifestations of fun are relatively easily explained, trying to say what fun feels like is not so straightforward. We are comfortable referring activities as fun, and when we do so we anticipate that the person we are telling will identify with a general affective state associated with having fun. We clearly have a sense of having fun, and most would concede that it feels distinct when we are having it from when we are experiencing other things. Quite how it feels when we are having fun is not easy to put into words. In the survey conducted for this study people were asked how fun differed from happiness or pleasure. As I shall illustrate later in the chapter many people resorted to the language of sensations to distinguish between these three phenomena—but when asked to describe how they *felt* having fun, in an embodied sense, people struggled. As a result I became interested in the question, if we have trouble identifying what fun is and what it feels like, how do we know we are having it? This chapter will go some way to exploring the sensational language of fun and suggest that we do know when we are having fun but have difficulty describing it. The interrelatedness of situation or context and the personal or psychological in creating conditions for fun make it very difficult to discern in any clear sense what the phenomenon is or

© The Editor(s) (if applicable) and The Author(s) 2016
B. Fincham, *The Sociology of Fun*,
DOI 10.1057/978-1-137-31579-3_6

what it feels like. It is much easier to rely on descriptions of activities that are commonly associated with fun, pointing, once again, to the social situatedness of something that is often referred to in naturalistic terms.

Early on in this project, I asked my partner to describe fun. Her answer was so good, I got her to repeat it and I wrote it down. What I like about it is that it touches many of the themes that make fun such an interesting topic. She said:

> [Fun is] a wonderful example of being in the moment. In *that* moment… why it's so lovely is because you are free in that moment and you are silly and you are disinhibited so you don't really have to think of it when you are having it. Free of that judgemental internal dialogue about 'should I, shouldn't I? Is it, isn't it? You're just there. I think that's one of the nicest things about it' (Bree Macdonald, June 2014)

In this quote Bree nods towards freedom, spontaneity, disinhibition, subjectivity, temporality, frivolity and sociality. The nowness of fun is clearly important, and, as has been pointed out elsewhere, temporality is a prominent feature of fun. Given this, it might be assumed that our feelings or sensations when we are in the moment are important too. However, the significance of the moment often becomes apparent in retrospect. In which case how fun feels in the moment becomes less important than the semantic attempt to faithfully communicate the sensations of having fun—particularly if the way of having fun is not universally experienced. Examples could be trainspotting, rugby or shopping, where, in order to communicate the fun to somebody that does not find these things fun requires a common language of experience that inevitably moves you away from sensate expression to the semantics of dialogue. Relatedly, we sometimes recast experiences in ways that are explicable to others but do not reflect the actual experience. As I have mentioned, cycling is a good example of this for me. I know I like it and I often tell people how much fun it is, but most of the time when I am doing it I would not say that I am having fun.

As has been indicated in the chapter on fun at work—fun is difficult to create, and in order to explain what it feels like requires a level of analysis, in the moment, that is antithetical to the experience of having fun. If you started thinking about how you were having fun and what it felt like when you were having it, you would stop having it.

Given these constraints it is not surprising that there is little written about what fun feels like and this is true for the sensual world more generally. Phenomenological or embodied descriptions are notoriously difficult due to the constraints of language—we simply don't have enough words to describe how we feel—but this does not mean that we don't acknowledge our phenomenal selves.

There are some that suggest that we have access to the 'being-in-the-world' outlined by Merleau-Ponty if only we could reorient ourselves to the sensual world. In order that we might get a sense of what having fun feels like phenomenologists would suggest that we need to shift the gaze towards the body as the main conduit for sense making. Pagis' study of meditation suggests that we have access to states of mind which enable phenomenal levels of analysis:

> The body is a 'mirror of our being'. By shifting attention to sensations in their bodies, meditators start sensing themselves sensing the world. They become aware of the somatic self, which consists of endless embodied feedback loops that are part of their beings. Such awareness can lead to interpretations and meaning-makings that take place in a discursive realm, as one engages in internal conversations, connecting bodily experiences to symbolic worlds of meaning. Yet if the body takes over and becomes the main channel for self-monitoring, a different mode of reflexivity is revealed. Here, self-to-self relations take place through the monitoring of the non-verbal meaning hidden in somatic images. By relaxing certain embodied responses and habitualizing new responses, a mediator can monitor his or her emotional and mental state. (Pagis 2009: 279)

Obviously, the meditative state and a state of having fun are different but the point that these things are experienced through the body is important. Fun is a social phenomenon and understood in relation to others, but it is not only experienced in interactional terms. At the times in which fun is had where we are, who we are with and what we feel define the experience. We have limited resources for analysing sentiments and sensations in moments in which we are having them. The different mode of reflexivity referred to by Pagis where the suggestion is that a person in the moment relaxes certain embodied responses and habitualises new responses points towards a mode of analysis where sensation and the sensual are put centre stage. Interestingly, when asked, many people identify this embodied experience, even in recollection. We have a sense of the experience of having fun that does not necessarily refer to its social nature. Perhaps this is best explained by Merleau-Ponty when he suggests:

> At the root of all our experiences and all our reflections, we find, then, a being which immediately recognizes itself… not by observation and as a given fact, nor by inference from any idea of itself, but through direct contact with that experience. (Merleau-Ponty 2002 [1945]: 232)

Fun does not hold up well under direct scrutiny. If a person thinks too hard about the fun they are having whilst they are having it the experience is changed, and plenty of people have told me that when I have asked them to analyse fun whatever it was stopped being fun. Merleau-Ponty represents 'direct contact' with experience as an unreflexive process. There is no space for reflexivity *about* fun during fun, that's just not how we experience it or how it works.

There are hints outside of academic literature highlighting the difficulty we have in describing how fun feels. There have been a couple of occasions where online forums have hosted the question what does fun feel like. One example was hosted on the online forum Storify. There is clearly a struggle here to adequately account for sensations—the respondents refer to lightness and love, descriptions equally as oblique as fun itself. One contributor said, 'I lose track of time, my spirit is light, I may be surprised and I may surprise myself' (Storify 2013) and another said, 'It's easy. Like light. Like love. Just easy' (Storify 2013). As will be demonstrated later, lightness and floating speak to the embodied experiences that are not well served by language. When these people are recollecting a sense of fun they are attempting to communicate the direct contact with the experience that Merleau-Ponty speaks of.

Another forum, hosted by Yahoo Answers, posed the question 'what does fun feel like to you?' Amongst the responses posted there were, 'Fun feels like a barrel of monkeys! Pleasure, mostly from the heart. My fun usually requires my brain as well, so generally speaking, fun for me is when I feel good all over!' Another said, 'To me it feels like being totally alive in the moment. Undistracted. Sometimes it is so absorbing I can only label it as fun after the fact!' (Yahoo Answers 2013).

There is obviously a problem of explaining what sensations feel like. We are often forced to use similes and metaphors, like lightness, like love, like floating, rather than being able to directly address the experience directly.

Can Focussing on Happiness Help Us Develop a Language for What Fun Feels Like?

A little less than I had hoped. Throughout the duration of this project on fun, happiness studies has run alongside, and whilst referring to these studies has been useful for some aspects of the study of fun, it has had limited utility in other areas. This is the case when it comes to understanding how best to analyse sensations in a social scientific way. I had imagined happiness studies would have a relatively sophisticated formula for doing this. And indeed people have written about how we feel when we are happy (Carr 2011; Csikszentmihalyi 2013; Catalino et al. 2014). Whilst some try, most of these sorts of sources do not account for how we sense or feel happiness. I was after analytic or even methodological tips as to how to express sensations in the moment—rather than observations about attentiveness or understanding the moment, for example. However, as early as in the eighteenth century it was acknowledged that the ethereal or amorphous nature of happiness made it difficult to capture. Kant refers to this in the *Groundwork to the Metaphysics of Morals* when he says:

> Unfortunately, the notion of happiness is so indeterminate that although every human being wishes to attain it, yet he [sic] can never say definitely and constantly what it is that he really wishes and wills.
> (Kant [1785] 2005: 78)

In a Kantian sense the inexplicability of happiness is a reflection of the nature of the phenomenon. We crave something that we cannot properly identify. At the same time we will all profess to periods of time that we would describe as happy or that we have experienced happiness even though we are unable to express what it is. This lack of certainty has persisted. In *The Second Sex* Simone de Beauvoir says, 'It is not too clear what the word happy means and still less what true values it may mask' (de Beauvoir [1949] 1974: 28). In the previous work on the discourse of the work/life balance, I have adopted the rather cynical stance iterated by de Beauvoir when it comes to well-being or happiness. It is mobilised for specific ends in specific contexts. This is not to suggest that we don't experience something that gives us feelings associated with happiness but that we should be suspicious of encouragements to it or definitions of it. Sara Ahmed observes, 'Happiness translates its wish into a politics, a wishful politics, a politics that demands others live according to a wish… the happy housewife is a fantasy figure that erases the signs of happiness' (Ahmed 2010: 2). For me this points to the idea that there is a construct at work at the same time as our experience of something—be that happiness or fun—that we assume are outside of social constructs or mediated definitions. We are supposed to just feel happiness, we are supposed to just have fun—but there are no straightforward ways of defining or understanding either.

This clearly relates to the moral imputation highlighted by Wolfenstein. Casting experiences that have no inherent properties as good or bad, as making us happy or unhappy, as fun or not fun requires a degree of social regulation. Ahmed, talking again about happiness, uses Locke to draw distinctions between *intentional* happiness and *affective* happiness. She suggests that intentional happiness is directed towards objects and is best understood in terms of 'I know that makes me happy because it has in the past' whereas affective happiness involves something like 'contact with [this thing] is making me happy' (Ahmed 2007: 124–5). There is clearly an interplay between the affective and the structural—just like anything else—and Ahmed's suggestion is that happiness is experienced in a relational way and this is the same for fun. When it comes to having fun we have an orientation towards experiences that will determine our feelings towards them and these work with expectations that are either confirmed or confounded. Understandings of what is fun and what is not fun are mediated by all sorts of social factors.

Despite this there are some that talk about experiences of happiness at least as intrinsic and deeply felt, in ways that cross cultural and temporal boundaries. For example, Mihaly Csikszentmihalyi, one of the early advocates of 'positive psychology, talks about 'flow' as an intrinsic psychological state which inspires responses in humans that transcend the social. He relates the story of a composer that he interviewed who described composing when its going well as inducing an 'ecstatic state' (Csikszentmihalyi 2004). As will be discussed a little later this relates to some extent to the sense of euphoria described by a couple of people that I spoke to about fun. Csikszentmihalyi describes how the composer becomes completely engrossed in the ecstatic moment:

> He doesn't have enough attention left over to monitor how his body feels, or his problems at home. He can't feel even that he's hungry or tired. His body disappears, his identity disappears from his consciousness, because he doesn't have enough attention, like none of us do, to really do well something that requires a lot of concentration, and at the same time to feel that he exists. So existence is temporarily suspended. And he says that his hand seems to be moving by itself. (Csikszentmihalyi 2004)

Csikszentmihalyi goes on to suggest that this is a universally experienced phenomenon:

> Now, when we do studies—we have, with other colleagues around the world, done over 8,000 interviews of people—from Dominican monks, to blind nuns, to Himalayan climbers, to Navajo shepherds—who enjoy their work. And regardless of the culture, regardless of education or whatever, there are… conditions that seem to be there when a person is in flow. There's this focus that, once it becomes intense, leads to a sense of ecstasy, a sense of clarity: you know exactly what you want to do from one moment to the other; you get immediate feedback. You know that what you need to do is possible to do, even though difficult, and sense of time disappears, you forget yourself, you feel part of something larger. And once the conditions are present, what you are doing becomes worth doing for its own sake. (Csikszentmihalyi 2004)

This sort of a-cultural standpoint is very seductive when it comes to thinking about happiness or fun generally, let alone with reference to embodied sensibilities. However, I am more cautious than

Csikszentmihalyi and find I am more closely aligned with people like Sara Ahmed, Stevi Jackson and Sue Scott. In their paper on the social construction of female orgasm, Jackson and Scott place naturalised embodied accounts squarely in court of social interaction:

> Sexual encounters arguably engender a greater sense of embodied selfhood than many other forms of social interaction, but it must be remembered that they are social. For it is here, especially when discussing desire and pleasure, that many theorists too easily fall back on understandings of the libidinal as fundamentally a property of the psyche, thus uprooting sexuality from social context. In contrast we set out to analyse embodied selves in socially located interaction. In focusing on sexual pleasure we consider how desire and pleasure may be reflexively understood in the context of everyday/everynight sexual practices. (Jackson and Scott 2007: 96)

For Jackson and Scott acknowledging the social embeddedness of a phenomenon does not deny its material manifestation—it simply places it as understood through the social contexts in which it is experienced. For me this is similar to fun. The dominant theme throughout this book is that fun is a social activity, but it is no less phenomenally experienced because of that.

'Please Try and Describe to Me What "Having Fun" Feels Like'

Particularly in the light of phenomenological observations, the data gathered for the survey on fun revealed much more sophisticated and imaginative ways of expressing a phenomenon that, like happiness, proved to be difficult to adequately describe.

The responses in the survey to the question 'please try and describe to me what "having fun" feels like' were rich and, I thought, often quite beautiful or uplifting. The first thing that struck me when analysing the data was that people had given the question proper consideration. As with data presented in other chapters, there is no easy way to disentangle the themes, many of which cross over and play with each other.

Initially I themed the data across behavioural, dis/embodied, ethereal, lack of self-consciousness and metaphorical categories, and they work for the most part—but most people talked across all of these themes, even in very few words. Organising them, whilst recognising the overlaps between them, exposes interesting features of the data.

Happiness

Happiness was the most recurrent theme in these data, but it was mentioned in relation to other things—relaxation, experiences, absorption and 'being in the moment' featured as present with happiness to create a situation that was fun. It could be that happiness is mentioned as a sort of stock response until something less oblique occurred to the respondent. One thing that became clear throughout the project was that people are unused to thinking in any great detail about fun. However, it is also the case that fun and happiness are often associated—one being the by-product of the other.

Happiness and …Relaxation

A persistent problem throughout my time with fun has been the automatic conflation of it with happiness, pleasure or any number of other positive affective states. However, when asked about how fun feels, many people talked about happiness as being a predicate of fun—it is a core component for many people. But what makes fun fun is happiness plus other factors—and these varied across a range of core themes. For some relaxation or feeling relaxed was an important component. One person suggested fun felt like 'A lightness of spirit, a [sic] openness to the world, a feeling of relaxation and happiness' (F29, Researcher) whilst another said 'Being happy and relaxed and really enjoying what you are doing' (F21, Student). Another student said 'you get this internal feeling of joy and happiness. You find yourself relaxing in the most cases and opening up to experiences' (M29, Student).

Happiness and Experiences

Several people associated happiness and experiences or activities as being the mechanism by which they understood themselves to be having fun. One person suggested 'an act that makes you extremely happy, feels like you don't want it to end, feeling of content [sic]' (F21, University student), whilst another student said:

> Being really happy/content. Smiling a lot. Being involved in an activity. I can be 'happy' alone, but when I have fun I'm either with people or doing something that engages mind and body. So I'd have to say that I think fun is quite a social phenomenon. It feels like you're enjoying and absorbed fully in the present moment. (F19, Student)

There is a lot going on in this quote. Happiness or contentedness is the bedrock of this person's sense of fun, but the combination of this positive affective state with active participation in something, sociality and being in absorbed in the moment combine to produce fun—this is interesting as it indicates that, whilst there is a sensual component to how this person experiences fun—smiling, contentedness—it is recognised without necessarily having to refer to these sensual components. Feelings of enjoyment are as socially mediated as any other—and for this person the social is particularly important in placing experiences as one thing or another.

Happiness, Absorption and 'Being in the Moment'

Many people identified absorption and what some described as 'being in the moment' as being part of the sensation of fun. It is a consistent conundrum for me as to how you know that you are distracted—by its definition a person would not be aware of being distracted; otherwise they wouldn't be distracted. However, several people identified a level of distraction as a component of how fun feels. One said, 'Fun is a happy, anxiety free feeling. It is being in the moment, being completely absorbed' (F48, Physical therapist), whilst another suggested 'having fun just feels like you are happy in the moment and even the negatives are outweighed'

(F20, Student). I think that the feeling of being in the moment amplifies the temporality of fun. Whilst it might sound tautological, the temporal boundedness of fun is highlighted by distraction from time. As a researcher said, fun feels like 'absorption in task, not worrying about anything else (yet sometimes awareness that this is a special time that will soon be over' (F32, Full-time academic researcher). We are able to accurately identify when fun stops when we are brought back from distraction—when we become aware of elements of situations or experiences that are not fun. These other elements do not have to be negative but they bring us into contexts that are not predicated by distraction. Related to distraction is a feeling of freedom; this will be further explored in a short while in the section on carefree fun, but several people identified freedom, specifically, in association with happiness as best to describe how fun feels. This couldn't be more explicitly explained than the student who said 'Happy feeling—free' (F22, Student). A lovely quote accentuating many aspect of freedom and the carefree nature of fun was provided by a TV director, who said that fun felt like

> a sense of being outside time, part of a process. Unselfconsciousness. A leaving behind of the normal day-to-day self and the usual worries. Often there's a sense of freedom and possibilities, of the world being a benign place. It's not always funny. But it usually makes you smile. It's relaxing, you feel kinder, more tolerant (though sometimes only after with sport). It involves other people and a feeling of connection with them. Of being known. (M44, Television producer/director)

This person identifies temporality, smiling, a connection with others and importantly freedom. I like the idea that part of fun for them is the opening up of possibilities and an activation of the world. Perhaps it is not particularly clever or rigorous analysis but this certainly resonates with my own conscious awareness of fun sometimes. There is a thrill about realising in the moment that other fun things are possible as a result of the fun currently being experienced. There is something about the unknowable consequences of abandonment that I, and these respondents, experience as fun.

Disinhibited and Carefree Fun

As I suggested, the crossovers in much of the data have made arranging them thematically difficult. Several of the comments above might as well have been coded to disinhibition and carefree attitudes; however, the contributions above all identified happiness and something else as how fun feels. In a similar way to the previous section there is a distinct lack of sensual or embodied accounts. I'm not entirely sure why this is aside from people being unused to giving embodied or sensual accounts of experiences that they have. There were a fair number of people that identified a specific type of distraction as a definitional characteristic of what fun feels like—namely, everyday concerns or anxieties as opposed to a distracted sense of time or task. As a lawyer suggested, a lack of attention to everyday concerns is synonymous with a carefree sensibility. They suggested fun is 'feeling happy, carefree, away from strains of everyday life, enjoying yourself there and then and thinking about it later and feeling good' (F48, Lawyer). I am not sure that this describes what fun feels like, other than 'good', but we do have visceral reactions to anxieties or concerns that are changed or not experienced when we are having fun. For some it appears as though fun felt like optimism in the face of current concerns, as a teacher said 'having fun feels like I don't have any anxieties and everything is going to be alright' (F34, Teacher at a Childcare Centre).

Others identified the carefree without being so explicit about it alleviating anything other than the humdrum. A PhD student said, 'Having fun is a happy feeling, and often involved laughing [sic] and smiling. It feels like freedom from mundane cares' (F33, PhD student). For many the escape from everyday worries is necessarily temporary—accentuating the temporal, as an occupational therapist said fun feels like 'enjoying the moment. Not wanting it to end. Light hearted. Usually amusing as well. Comfortable. Having fun distracts from more serious matters' (F36, Occupational therapist). As has been and will be further noted lightness or weightlessness is a consistent feature of these accounts. It is interesting that metaphorically speaking worries or concerns are often described as weighing heavy on people—so it is no surprise that distraction from these heavy matters induces descriptions of lightness from people.

This was summed up well by an IT engineer. In response to the question 'can you tell me what fun feels like?' he said:

> I'll try… Fun is freedom of thought. While having fun you are not concerned with the consequences, not concerned with the world outside of the activity that you are having fun doing. Fun will cause you to lose track of time, to forget that meeting tomorrow with the boss or the fact that you just broke up with your girlfriend. (M29, IT engineer)

Carefree Fun and Forgetting

Others described fun as feeling like a process of short-term forgetting. 'It feels like you can completely forget about everything you normally worry about. You're very much in the moment' (F21, Student and part-time sales assistant). Another person said, 'Having fun is temporarily forgetting things that are bothering you and focusing on activities that you have come to enjoy or that look appealing to you in some way. It is the thrill you get from such activities that let you know you're having fun' (F18, Student). It is worth noting that this explicit association with activities was relatively rare. Most agreed that activity, whilst a component, was not what made fun—as quoted earlier, Blythe and Hassenzahl's observation that 'a ride on a roller coaster can be enjoyable, but maybe not after an enormous dinner' (Blythe and Hassenzahl 2004: 94) is apposite at this juncture.

For some the relationship between a carefree time and a sensation is that is associated with the beneficial effects of having fun. An administrator said fun felt like 'forgetting any worries. Releasing your emotions. Feeling carefree. Feeling happy and that life is good' (F48, Admin person) whilst a law lecturer pointed out the role of transcendence in fun from activity:

> If you have responsibilities, you don't feel that you have them at that moment. You are living in the moment. What you are doing is important (some things are more likely to be fun than others), but fun transcends the activity (M49, Law lecturer)

This is an important observation. This person makes the association between being in the moment and transcendence from task. There is a general consensus that activity is not enough—things are not inherently fun, the participant has to be oriented towards an activity or sensation as fun, but quite how this works was not really explored by any respondents to the survey. The idea of transcendence from task or activity towards an orientation to it as positive and affective may help explain how things become fun. In a similar vein one person suggested that fun felt like 'carelessness, freedom from constraints, hedonism'. In a philosophical sense hedonism implies the pursuit of pleasure as a good. However, it is reasonable to anticipate that this person is suggesting that the freedom from constraints creates the space for having pleasure. Whilst not strictly speaking transcendent, it implies the orientation towards experiences that maximise positive effects away from sensibilities that inhibit positive effects.

Carefree Fun and a Lack of Self-Consciousness

For some people that responded to the survey the idea of a lack of self-consciousness was an important component that sat alongside a carefree sensibility and is then experienced. This is a specific orientation to being carefree that concentrates more on the self than on broader situational contexts. Once again the people that mentioned the abandonment of self-consciousness did so amongst many other things. For one person, spontaneity and experiences are allied with a lack of self-consciousness:

> Fun is not thinking how you're being perceived by others and not feeling self-conscious, feeling confident and not thinking about how 'good' you are at what you're doing. Also just enjoying yourself in a very simple way, perhaps spontaneously, like a kind of optimal experience maybe. (F26, Proofreader)

People tended to talk about conditions that inspire feelings that are associated with fun, rather than describing the sensation of having fun. A writer suggested that fun felt like a lack of self-consciousness and a sense of connectedness, for the it is 'a sense of rightness, of not being self-conscious, of being tuned in to nature or other people, of rediscovering the innocent fun of childhood' (F66, Writer). On a slightly different tack a student in the South East said fun felt like 'a sense of ease, where thoughts that bother you in the everyday world no longer inhibit your thoughts/behaviour and feelings. It's when you can just let go and enjoy where you are and who you are with' (M35, Student). It is interesting that for the last two people the lack of self-consciousness is experienced as fun when connected with others. It is the ease with others and the self that are important here. I think that this relates to a lack of inhibition related and a lack of feeling judged. This also accentuates that consistent point that for most people fun is a social affair. That said, enjoyment is, of course, important, 'I think it [is] where you enjoy yourself without being self-conscious of doing so' (M30, Lecturer).

Carefree Fun and Connectedness to Others

For several respondents this sense of connectedness of people was what occurred to them when asked what fun felt like. Other people do not necessarily define the experience but certainly appear to orient it in particular ways. I really like the combination of elements that were highlighted by a student in Brighton: 'Excitement, sense of community/feeling of belonging, not thinking about anything beyond the current situation' (F20, Student). For them excitement, connectedness with other people and temporality or the moment conspire to provoke the sensation of having fun, in a similar vein another student said fun feels 'like letting go, connecting with people, and letting your hair down' (F23, Student). For another person the closeness of relationships appears to be important: fun feels like 'carefree, stress free, time doing something interesting with friends or family' (F58, Professor and Head of Department).

A couple of respondents associated a carefree attitude to childhood, and the associated sensations. An outreach worker said that

> there is an element of abandon to having fun, a release that lets go of tensions and worries. For me, having fun involves an element of silliness and reverting to childhood so fun tends to be taking pleasure in fairly simple things. It feels like you are lighter and less serious a person. (F27, Outreach worker)

As was suggested in the chapter *Childhood and Fun* there is normally an automatic association with childhood and silliness or triviality. Given the number of people in the survey that mentioned temporary alleviation from serious anxieties or concerns this response is not surprising. What is a surprise to me is that so few people mentioned feeling like a child when asked what fun feels like—aside from the children that returned the survey, as they have nothing to compare 'feeling like a child' to anything else. Four other people that mentioned childhood said fun feels 'like being a kid again. Not feeling concerned or stressed in any way' (F27, Teacher).

Embodied Sensations

In asking the question 'can you tell me what fun feels like?' I had naively anticipated responses that would refer to sensations experienced by the body that let people know that they are having fun. As has been illustrated this was not the case in most of the responses. People seem to be more comfortable describing the conditions that will provoke a set of sensations that can be interpreted as having fun. In subsequent conversations with friends, particularly in Café & Salvage in Hove (a very good café if you find yourself in Hove, and where much of this book was written), it turns out that articulating sensations for a phenomena that is itself pretty amorphous is more difficult than one might have anticipated. As will be explored later, I think this is largely because we are not aware of having fun when we are having it. We tend to apply the label of fun to some experiences post hoc in order to make them explicable to ourselves, and others, as a particular type of positive experienced in the past and understood in the present. What those positive experiences actually consist of, however, is not entirely clear.

That said, about a quarter of the respondents (28%) did refer to sensations that I am interpreting as descriptions of embodied responses of one type or another to varying degrees. Some referred to a general sense of being alive when having fun. A person in Dublin associated this alive feeling with activity and contentedness, saying, 'Having fun feels like happiness, and liveliness, even if it's just reading a book, you feel a bit more alive or content' (F31, PhD student), whilst another highlighted the role of distraction that works, for them, alongside a heightened sense of being alive: 'It's very unique. It's basically happiness. You feel energized and active. Your attention is focussed and it isn't a chore to do so' (M19, Student). For these two people there is an interesting effect of having fun as concentrating attention to the moment and to the body. Another person suggested 'having fun makes me feel happy and has a general calming, soothing [sic] affect' (M47, Controller/CFO). Whilst it could be contended that this is not a strictly embodied response I think that the deployment of the term soothing suggests something more than a calming of the mind. These kinds of responses are general in their reference to embodied responses to fun. Others were more specific.

Laughter and Smiling

By a country mile the most common response that involved a bodily sensation or reaction to having fun was smiling and/or laughing. Whilst it could be argued that this is not a sensation in itself, my sense is that there is something universalisable in laughter as a sensual experience. Bearing in mind that the question that was asked was, 'Please try and describe to me what having fun feels like' the responses that invoked smiling or laughing are interesting because of the thought that smiling or laughing feels like something. Many of the responses were simple and straightforward, for example, 'Feeling like you are going to laugh, but not at a joke' (M49, University lecturer) and 'It makes you want to laugh and smile' (F43, Lecturer). Thirteen people mentioned laughing as the key component of having fun, with five of those people suggesting that it is the combination of laughing with relaxation that best describes what fun feels like. Amongst these responses involving laughter people mentioned 'A high, a buzz' (F50, Part-time lecturer) and an inability to stop laughing (F39, Academic). These two responses relate to the lack of inhibition and joyous abandonment that others identified as components of having fun. Another person identified the temporal element in having fun saying fun feels like 'any transient moment that makes me grin or laugh for awhile' (F59, Plant area manager in a garden centre). For others laughter was not mentioned but another facial response—smiling—was. As the student from Bath in an earlier quote suggested that smiling and fun were synonymous in their mind with social interaction.

The combination of sociality, temporality and the related being in the moment, absorption and smiling are accentuated. Here the distinction between this person's understanding between happiness and fun is important—for her the social aspect of positive, happy, absorbed, smiley times is fun. These conditions are not prerequisites for happiness. It has become clear throughout the project that the social is a key characteristic of fun—and for me this is summed up in the schema of fun (Chap. 2) in a relationship to interaction. There is an interactional element to understanding and communicating fun that is to do with others—shared experiences, communicating experiences or knowing that others will understand experiences as fun. I'm not sure that I would go as far as suggesting that this is just a question of construct as I do think that sensations of positivity are felt, but as any symbolic interactionist will tell you social construct is always writ large in any social interaction. Another respondent highlighted the role of connection in being a characteristic in how fun feels:

> It can be many different experiences. Laughing with others not least when sharing common experience. Achieving something, often when it's a little scary and just enjoying a beautiful experience whether it is nature or another human being. (M66, Consultant)

I very much like this quote. Fun can be beautiful aesthetically, emotionally, sensually, messily, spontaneously and euphorically—perhaps this a vernacular foible but I think of the word beautiful when I think of how fun feels. For the previous respondent the connectedness of experiencing fun is not just limited to humans, but they also suggest that a connection with nature creates conditions for feeling fun and laughter. Another person picked up on the social component but also accentuates the embodied element with the idea of tension and release. For her fun feels like 'something slightly decadent, enjoyed between a few people, silly, funny. Physical release of tension with laughter' (F33, Facilities co-ordinator). Decadence, irreverence and naughtiness are themes that have been picked up elsewhere, but it is interesting that this person associates decadence with a feeling or sensation.

Lightness

It was interesting that many people mentioned lightness or weightlessness as a phenomenal experience to describe fun. Perhaps it is obvious, but it hadn't occurred to me that it would feature as often as it did. Levity and joy are often associated with sayings such as 'lightness of heart' so maybe it shouldn't be a surprise that it is used to describe feelings and sensations associated with levity, joy and fun. Alongside lightness an IT manager in London mentioned effortlessness; for them fun feels like 'heightened levels of brain activity with a total lack of intellectual effort and a lightness of being' (M35, Go-getter rock star party animal/IT manager). For some a lack of effort is important to understanding the role of fun in a life that is often quite hard work. If fun is a temporary alleviation from the stresses of everyday life—often defined through effort—then fun should not be an effort. You cannot really work hard to have fun, that's not how it happens. As a young woman in Brighton says fun feels like 'not worrying about things you would usually worry about. Feeling light and weightless' (F20, Student). Another student suggests that the lightness is felt—and the experience of laughing and lightness are located firmly in the sensual body. For them fun feels like 'laughing in an uninhibited way, and a light feeling in my chest' (F44, Student). This lightness is felt in particular ways for some respondents. I like the way in which fizzing and bubbling were mentioned by people as visceral experiences and by way of a link to the next section I have placed the following two quotes at the end of this section: one saying that fun feels like 'lightness, absence of worry, bubbly feeling, feeling comfortable and present in my body' (Trans22, Student); another suggesting it is 'lightness in the chest; fizzy feeling in your veins; floaty' (F43, Part-time researcher and full-time mother to toddler twins).

Giggly, Bubbly and Fizzy

As with the previous two excerpts there were people that described feelings in terms commonly associated with excitement. The fizzy feeling in the veins described by the researcher is an effective way of describing an embodied sensation but also highlights the paucity of words available to us to describe positive sensations. Others that used similar language said fun felt like 'a mix between feeling happy and bubbly' (M19, Student), 'giggly inside and carefree' (F39, Teacher) and 'it feels warm, it makes you fizz!' (F52). I feel as though these sorts of descriptions relate to a sense of euphoria or intense excitement that provokes the fizzing, bubbling sensations.

Warmth

A surprising regular descriptor was warmth. For some of the respondents that used warmth to express what fun feels like there is a sense that fun brings comfort and joy. The combinations of descriptions that are used alongside warmth are also interesting. A student said fun feels like a 'sense of happiness and warmth inside. And just having a profound positive outlook on life. Smiling as well' (F19, Student). Whilst this person is describing conditions that can facilitate fun having, they are also drawing on embodied responses—smiling and warmth. A lecturer in the southwest of England said:

> I think fun is generally a short-term experience, and is comparable to a feeling. It is experienced when we do pleasurable activities, and I think fun often involves laughter. It is like a burst of pleasure that can make you feel warm inside. (F31, Lecturer)

They identify the temporal element of fun—it is bound in time, but they also associate it with activities. Fun is had when something is being done and the description of a 'burst of pleasure' speaks to a sort of ballistic response to situations that turn into fun. The recurrent theme of distraction from everyday concerns was expressed alongside warmth by an administrator when they said 'it gives you a warm glowing feeling inside, and makes me forget about my issues' (F40, Administrator). Just to accentuate the interconnectedness of all of these elements that people have identified one person said this, 'at its best, it involves a warm, elated feeling in the chest and light-headedness. Usually it involves laughter' (M22, Student). They have managed to incorporate many facets of fun identified by a number of other people—warmth, elation, lightness, laughter and sensations in the body.

Elation and Euphoria

It is interesting to me that more people did not mention elation or euphoria—although some did. I think that in euphoria many of the attendant features of fun that people had identified are present. Distraction from normality, absorption in the moment, often experienced with others and is experienced as a sensation located within the body. Perhaps if I had the chance to ask follow-up questions this would have been something I would have asked. As it goes I have had many subsequent conversations with people where I have asked about euphoria. Whilst most have agreed that it is present in lots of fun having, several have questioned whether it is a prerequisite for having fun, and that there are too many other sensations that can inform us about fun having. A couple of respondents to the survey simply wrote a single word, 'elation' (M56, Oil company executive), 'euphoric' (M37, Researcher), whilst others expanded:

> Having fun makes me feel giggly, and like I'm in a state of hysteria. I can feel quite giddy and euphoric. It can be quite an exhilarating experience, which you notice afterwards when you are calming down. (F21, Checkout assistant)

Whilst a lecturer said:

> It feels lights, it feels giddy, it makes me feel alive. And I can feel it right through my body. It makes me feel lifted, it is a real high. And it is a high I can revisit… as it lingers after the 'event' and I can remember it with a smile later on… probably for years (hopefully) (F47, Overworked Lecturer)

These last two comments, as with others, incorporate several previously mentioned and are suffused with excitement. They are also describing an experience rooted in the body. I relate to the idea of fun as an exhilarating experience. Mentions of highs, buzzes and rushes also point towards to sensual excitation as being a facet of how fun feels. I am aware that for some these descriptions will be mapped onto an essentialist biological body—one full of endorphins and adrenaline—and whilst they may be accurate portrayals of chemical reactions in the body they are less interesting to me than the feeling or sensations they produce. I prefer to interpret a high or a buzz in a socio-emotional way than a matter of the release of hormones into the bloodstream. Having said that several people did refer to the feeling of having fun in those terms.

Veins, Hearts and Adrenal Glands

It may seem perverse to bemoan the fact that everybody did not refer to actual sensations, but rather described conditions that provide the possibility for sensing fun, and then be sniffy about those that referred to organs or body parts; in suggesting that I prefer to think of having fun in socio-emotional terms does not mean that the sorts of embodied descriptions provided by some do not speak to that socio-emotional experience. For example, a school student said fun feels like 'a happiness inside of your heart that makes joyfulness pass through your veins which you can then express by simply smiling' (M14, High School student), and I love this description. It is conveys the joy and excitement that you feel in your body when you are having fun—it is sensed, experienced, *had* in a number of terrains—emotional, psychic, social, bodily. 'A mixture of happiness and adrenaline is how I see it' (M20, Student). Once again there is a relationship between the corporeal and the emotional. I do not think that references to the heart or the chest are metaphorical. There are occasions where the heart rate is heightened or you feel a swelling in the chest: 'Having fun to me is like a balloon being blown up in the middle of your chest you can feel it building and it's anticipation about how far the situation will go!' (F41, Vocational learning manager). The sense of anticipation described by the previous person implies an excitement that is physically manifest. The idea of seeing how far a situation will go also speaks to the immediacy of the experience, and whilst this person suggests that they are anticipating the (very near) future it is an excitement felt in the present. The heart is important to many affective descriptions, both positive and negative, and descriptions of fun are no different. As a person in Sussex said when describing what fun feels like, 'it brings joy to your heart and a smile to your face. It makes you forget your worry [sic] and cares for a while. It recharges your batteries and enables you to deal with the daily humdrum' (F47, Without work). For them fun connects an internal embodied sensation with an external manifestation—a smile—and also incorporates the nowness of the experience as well as the distraction.

Language and Bodies

There is an inherent problem with the language available to describing embodied experiences happiness and, I would argue, fun. So it should come as no surprise that people struggle with describing what fun feels like. On the whole I think that people did fairly well, but there was a propensity to describe the conditions that create the sensual experiences of fun or what fun actually feels like. As has been previously noted, I think this is largely to do with the fact that we are very rarely in a position to analyse embodied sensations in the moment. Stopping having fun in order to try and describe what it feels like is a bit like chasing your tail. Unless the fun is being had analysing how fun feels there is little opportunity to understand what we are feeling. This inexplicability means that descriptions are heavily reliant on metaphor and simile. In these linguistic devices we then anticipate that others will recognise this abstracted description of what things feel like. As we are not used to iterating our embodied sensations, we resort to a language of inferences and 'you know what I mean'. When it comes to fun, this is to do with the near impossibility of describing it whilst it is happening. As has been suggested earlier, the distracted nature of having fun means that as soon as attention is directed too closely to what is being experienced it stops being distracted—and consequently becomes something other than fun. However, this is not always the case. During a conversation with a friend she said that there are moments when you are aware and those moments are euphoric and overtly social. She described dancing at a club with a friend and them both grabbing each other and shouting that they were having a great time at each other. In that moment there is awareness that what is being *felt* is fun. In those moments what was described spoke very much to the connectedness of the people having fun, rather than what the body felt like.

Conclusion

The question of what fun feels like is interesting for a number of reasons. It is difficult to disentangle the phenomenal experience from assumptions about what we imagine it is supposed to feel like. There are very few occasions when we can recognise and then take account of how we are feeling at the moments in which we are having fun. Also, there is the problem of universalising, through language, our own subjective experiences. The analytic challenges in embodied research are known and not particularly well developed. This study is no exception, and at a later date I intend to start developing projects that can develop methods for analysing distracted states of consciousness sociologically. However, in a purely descriptive sense there were clear demarcations between metaphorical descriptions, activity-based descriptions and descriptions of embodied feelings in the data presented here. There is also the question of how we represent visceral experiences linguistically more generally. In terms of how fun was represented to me in response to the question 'tell me what fun feels like' the theme of happiness as an unproblematic description of a feeling rapidly emerged. There were many people that made the association between fun and happiness in conjunction with something else. So happiness and relaxation, happiness and absorption and happiness and experiences all featured as attempts by people to get at a way of expressing their fun to others—in this case me. As was mentioned towards the beginning of the chapter, it became clear that people had never really thought about what fun was or how it felt to any depth until I asked them. The association between fun and happiness is assumed rather than necessarily experienced. The sociality of fun, as opposed to happiness, was expressed—the thought being that it is possible to be happy alone but almost always we have fun with others. The theme of distraction within happiness was also identified as important. However, as with many of the other themes that were identified in the data, people tended to talk about circumstances or contexts in which they experienced fun, rather than what it actually felt like—even when pushed people found it difficult to conceptualise embodied sensations away from social contexts, circumstances or situations.

Some felt as though disinhibition, carefree or anxiety-free moments were central to their experience of fun. In a sense the lack of anxiety does speak to an embodied sensation—but this is the description of an absence of some feelings, rather than the presence of some. Once again this is more about the contexts within which fun happens—when a person is not focussed on their current concerns or anxieties they are more open to having fun.

There was a clearer sense of embodied reactions in the descriptions of laughter and smiling—this is a direct physical reaction to situations, and is also easily recognisable to others. In some of the data that mentioned laughter with others there is a clear reciprocity in the situation. This may also have echoes of Podilchak's condition for having fun—namely, the levelling out of power inequalities between people having the fun. Laughing hard and loud in the moment with others requires mutual understanding—the extent to which this is actually invested in parity, however, is a moot point. For some the freedom to laugh involved a level of disinhibition, so this embodied response is folded back into the socio-structural world where the interrelatedness of these elements of life becomes evident. In order to feel disinhibited you have to know the rules of inhibition, the flouting of these rules creates conditions where laughing with abandon become a possibility. It is then the case that we reframe this situation as a naturalistic or automatic reaction to a situation, person or relationship.

The descriptions that incorporated ideas of lightness and warmth were where respondents attempted to address the more sensational aspects of fun. In these accounts there was a connection between an embodied sensibility and a language that might adequately sum up how these moments feel. They are caught between visceral descriptions and the metaphorical. There are elements of both in attempts to capture experiences using lightness or warmth. In both there were many elements folded together. There is the phenomenal feeling of light-headedness, sometimes giddiness, but also a lightness of heart, a sensation of a lifting in the chest without effort. The idea of being warm inside or glowing is a common description of contentment or happiness, and I would debate the extent to which it is just a metaphor. It is part of the lexicon of happiness where a phenomenal experience is given a name that is not in itself accurately descriptive, and that then comes to mean that experience—in the loosest sense, a Weberian ideal type. When it comes to both lightness and warmth most of us understand what that feels like and those two words are the closest we have to describing the phenomenon. Related to warmth and lightness is euphoria. In the data, the mention of warmth and particularly lightness accompanied descriptions of intense or heightened emotional states. It occurs to me that this is a particular type of fun that involves bursts of energy and adrenaline. The intensity in the descriptions of this experience of fun was expressed are suffused with joy and elation.

The problems that many people had in describing what fun feels like is not surprising given how we experience fun as distracted and also how we experience it as a social phenomenon. As has been pointed out, it is antithetical to fun to concentrate on how you are experiencing it in the moment. By its nature fun involves attention being taken away from the phenomenal experience of it. The second confounding feature is that the question 'what does fun feel like?' directs attention towards the self where the phenomenon is experienced with reference to others. It is difficult to then characterise something that is felt subjectively but is not intrinsically derived and maintained. Fun is a social interaction that is determined by relationships and circumstances that are then experienced as fun. The ways in which it is then felt is with reference to the situation not necessarily the phenomenal feelings it inspires. A key finding of this book, and one that I had not previously considered, is that rather than understanding fun as underpinned by feelings it is supported and maintained by social relations—we recognise it socially and then represent it affectively.

The next chapter discusses the relationship between post hoc characterisations of experiences as fun, but this is clearly associated with our understandings or comprehension of the present, and implicit in this situation is embodied sensibilities. We experience the world in the moment through our bodies, but our attention is rarely directed towards it. However, the problem of describing what fun feels like is as much to do with assumptions we make about how we experience the world in relation to moments, as it is a question of vocabulary or semantics.

References

Ahmed, S. (2007). Multiculturalism and the promise of happiness. *New Formations, 63*, 121–137.

Ahmed, S. (2010). *The promise of happiness*. Durham: Duke University Press.

Blythe, M., & Hassenzahl, M. (2004). The semantics of fun: Differentiating enjoyable experiences. In M. Blythe, K. Overbeeke, A. Monk, & P. Wright (Eds.), *Funology: From usability to enjoyment*. London: Kluwer.

Carr, A. (2011). *Positive psychology: The science of happiness and human strengths*. London: Routledge.

Catalino, L., Algoe, S., & Fredrickson, B. (2014). Prioritizing positivity: An effective approach to pursuing happiness. *Emotions, 14*(6), 1155–1161.

Csikszentmihalyi, M. (2004, February). Flow: The secret to happiness. *TEDtalk*. http://www.ted.com/talks/mihaly_csikszentmihalyi_on_flow. Accessed 24 Oct 2015.

Csikszentmihalyi, M. (2013). *Flow: The psychology of happiness*. London: Rider.

de Beauvoir, S. (1974[1949]). *The second sex*. New York: Vintage.

Jackson, S., & Scott, S. (2007). Faking it like a woman? Towards an interpretative theorisation of sexual pleasure. *Body and Society, 13*(2), 95–116.

Kant, I. ([1785] 2005). *Groundwork for the metaphysics of morals*. Toronto: Broadview Publishing.

Merleau-Ponty, M. (2002 [1945]). *Phenomenology of perception*. London: Routledge.

Pagis, M. (2009). Embodied self-reflexivity. *Social Psychology Quarterly, 72*(3), 265–283.

7

Fun and Recollection

As has been illustrated in the previous chapter, there are relationships between the experiences or sensations of having fun in the moment and our retelling or reconstruction of experiences as fun. The example of cycling is, in my experience, illustrative of a reconstructive process. I have often been riding with friends where I have found the ride tough. Struggling up Ditchling Beacon in Sussex, wishing I were anywhere else in the world and feeling as though I want to pass out or throw up or both. However, these moments of discomfort and unhappiness swiftly fade as the summit is crossed and the ride becomes easier. In the pub, sometime after the ride, my friends and I will agree that today's ride was great fun, the scenery was beautiful and that it is very good to get out on your bike. In fact, I catch myself telling all sorts of people how much fun it is to ride a bike—particularly to those that don't really like cycling—but when I think about it, whilst I think I like it in the moment, I rarely have fun. I think it is the same with many activities assumed to be fun. That is not to say that people are not enjoying such activities; it's just that there is a post hoc application of the status of fun to certain activities in order to make them explicable in positive terms to others. Fun offers not only positivity but also a lightness to the expression of experiences, and this narrative need not necessarily reflect how the thing being experienced actually felt.

Alongside a narrative of 'fun' making sense of recent experiences, it also relates to feelings or sentiments that echo over time, the relationship to childhood experiences and fun is strong—as has been illustrated elsewhere in the book. This also manifests in views of fun as childish—in both negative and positive ways.

So, there is a question of the points at which fun is experienced. As will be discussed, there is something about the role of memory and recollection in reconstituting a recent past that needs interrogating with regard to how fun is professed and the extent to which we construct fun or apply the status of fun to events or experiences post hoc. Many of the events or experiences described in studies are retold as fun. Once again this raises issues of temporality and the question of the extent to which a narrative provides templates for understanding experiences as one thing or another but often after the experience has finished. In this chapter I am not suggesting that fun is entirely a figment of a reimagined past. What is argued is that memory and recollection play an important role in what we think is fun and how we have it.

Memories and Positive Experiences in the Present

Bryant, Smart and King published a paper in the *Journal of Happiness Studies* in 2005 where they say that 'positive reminiscing' serves a specific role in casting the present in a positive light (Bryant et al. 2005). In this paper they suggest that, at the time of their writing, concentration on positive reminiscing focussed on the experiences of older people (Bryant et al. 2005: 228), and much of the academic output of that time discusses remembering as generally directed towards producing therapeutic outcomes for older age care (Einstein et al. 1992; Mather and Carstensen 2005; Schlagman et al. 2006). Of interest to considerations of fun is the demonstration of casting back in order to explain the present. They acknowledge the long-held belief that reminiscence plays a role in identity formation and identity maintenance (Bryant et al. 2005: 228). Bryant, Smart and King then go on to talk about the role of positive reminiscence in younger people—where the focus of study is away from directly therapeutic outcomes and towards meanings that this tendency might foster. They quote research from Pasupathi and Carstensen, which incorporated data from both the young and old, where it was found 'social reminiscing was an effective emotion regulation strategy in enhancing positive emotions' (Bryant et al. 2005: 229). From their own findings Bryant, Smart and King say:

> Our results suggest that the adaptive value of reminiscence is not so much a form of escape from present problems, but rather as a constructive tool for increasing awareness and providing a sense of perspective for the present. (Bryant et al. 2005: 236)

Whilst Pasupathi and Carstensen and Bryant, King and Smart are understanding reminiscing as a particular type of remembering I think that it is useful in suggesting that a particular orientation to the recent past—even something that has only just happened—can determine not just how we feel in the present but how we assume we felt in the past. In a discursive sense the reconstitution of the past into something meaningful to ourselves and also explicable to others is very important for establishing a narrative of experiences but also, as is acknowledged by Bryant, Smart and King, is important for identity. As has been mentioned elsewhere, particularly in relation to fun morality, how we demonstrate our fun impacts on how others view us, and also establishes criteria by which we understand our own positive experiences. Of course this does not simply impact on a sense of the self. How we have fun also determines with whom we have fun—people that enjoy each other's company socialise together. Alongside the individual narratives that are constructed by the deployment of memories or reminiscences there is also a broader social role in that the individual narratives need to make sense to a wider social sphere. As has been illustrated throughout this book, our experiences of fun are fairly narrowly defined—people tend to have fun in remarkably similar ways, despite it being characterised as very subjective.

Halbwachs and the Reconstruction of the Past

In his writing on memory and recall Maurice Halbwachs offers a method for interpreting the echoes from childhood as present and interpretable in adulthood.

> When one of the books which were the joy of our childhood, which we have not opened since, falls into our hands, it is not without a certain curiosity, an anticipation of a recurrence of memories and a kind of interior rejuvenation that we begin to read it. Just by thinking about it we believe that we can recall the mental state in which we found ourselves at that time. (Halbwachs 1992: 46)

For Halbwachs there is an interesting relationship between memory and a sense of the past. Whilst we may have vague recollections of events or people, particularly from our childhood, we tend to have strong impressions of childhood. We can summon up an overall feeling of what it was like to be a child in situations—and often these are very strong feelings. Halbwachs continues with the rediscovered book, 'We therefore hope by reading the book again to complete the former vague memory and so to relive the memory of our childhood' (Halbwachs 1992: 46). For this sense of the past to resonate throughout our lives Halbwachs suggests that we 'preserve' memories from parts of our lives and that these are continually reproduced. It is in this process that 'a sense of our identity is perpetuated' (Halbwachs 1992: 47). I would suggest that it is not just identity that is perpetuated but also our own unique orientations to phenomena. So the interior rejuvenation that Halbwachs talks about includes reacting to things on the basis of how we have previously reacted to things. When it comes to fun, consistently reporting enjoyment, or deriving fun, through mechanisms that we have developed through our lifetimes, perpetuates the sense of coherence in identity. I say unique orientations because of the myriad influences on us through our lives that determine, to a large extent, how we have fun, or what we experience as fun. These are many and varied. From upbringing, and family, to peers and schooling, from cultural sensibilities to micro interactions and relationships, we invent our own versions of fun. These follow broadly similar patterns but there is variance between people even in very similar circumstances. Social class has been identified as a filter through which people have in the past understood their happiness and pleasure (Phillips 1969; Collet-Sabe and Tort 2015) and it is reasonable to assume that this is also a factor in how we understand our own fun making—indeed as Blythe and Hassenzahl point out, the etymology of the word 'fun' is deeply classed. However, social class, for example, should not be taken as a simple determinant of how people have fun—it may be part of the story but other variables are influential. Many of us will have had the experience of going to a friend's house and being exposed to some game or interaction that the friends' family find great fun but that you find at best not much fun and at worst embarrassing. As we are growing up it is noticeable how types of fun diverge between groups of children that are growing up together. Some find physical games fun, others find more sedentary activities fun. Reading is fun for some and not for others; drawing, climbing, being 'naughty', skateboarding, playing war games, music, all divide children in various directions all influenced by things—and norms and messages—that surround them. This is a fairly standard account of socialisation—nothing wrong with that—and what it points to is the idea that our orientations towards things are not formed through individual instances of experiencing them but through general exposure to the influences that determine how we are expected to react to those things. If this is the case, then where does it leave childhood memories of fun? I think it is generally assumed that we are aware of when we had fun in childhood, because we can remember it. I suppose this may be so for some people, but as is obvious from the direction of this chapter, I am drawn to Halbwachs' summary of what adults do with their idea of their own childhoods. We preserve memories and reproduce them so that our identity and sense of our selves are perpetuated and this seems normal because of the distractions of everyday life, so with reference to identity Halbwachs says:

> It seems fairly natural that adults, absorbed as they are with everyday preoccupations. Is it not the case that adults deform their memories of childhood precisely because they force them to enter the framework of the present? (Halbwachs 1992: 47)

I don't think that Halbwachs is suggesting that we don't have memories; rather, these memories are deployed in the present to support particular aspects of identity in relation to a personal history. The memories that are deployed in social settings do work for us. When it comes to fun, it can be to accentuate our distance from that stage of life, for instance, 'it used to be fun but is not anymore' or to accentuate the coherence between stages of life and our sense of self, for instance, 'I've always found that fun.' This does raise the question of childish play. As adults we appear to have an ambivalent relationship to childish play often regretting its passing or attempting to manufacture an adult version of it—but rarely simply enjoying it with the lack of inhibition or self-consciousness that we associate with childhood, until we become old, according Halbwachs. In older age we are less self-conscious when it comes to childish types of play because we are less likely to have to behave in a way that demonstrates seriousness or responsibility. According to Halbwachs, there is a difference between society, as we live it in the present, and the imagined society in which we immerse ourselves when we remember—he suggests, 'We choose from the past the period in which we wish to immerse ourselves.' In this case our memory of having fun is located in an imagined past and we are instrumental in creating the ambience and even the setting of our memories. We use the reference points that are available to us in order to then reconstruct a sense of a time gone by. For me there is great potency in the memories that I have of playing the football game Subbuteo[1] in my bedroom aged about nine, with the sun streaming through my window. In my recollection I can feel the heat of the sun, can smell my room and have a palpable sense of the contentment and fun that I was having. However, if I were asked when that was, which teams I had playing, what I did next or at what point did I think that this form of fun ceased for me I would not be able to answer. My parents have photographs of my brother and me in our childhood; these props are useful for augmenting the apparent accuracy of my memories. There is also the suspicion that I have no authentic memories of many of the occasions captured by my father's camera, but have documentary

---

[1] Professional football at your fingertips!

evidence and the associated narratives woven by the family about what happened and how we felt in these places and times. Halbwachs suggests that memory gives us the illusion of living in the midst of groups which do not imprison or constrain us. In our memories we are unfettered by the *actuality* of a situation—we can sense it as being better or worse or different than we might have experienced it—and this is possible because of the perspectival element of memories attributed to individuals and because of the necessity to identity of shoehorning memories into forms that fit with the present. That present consists not only of our selves but also of the social contexts that shape expectations and, according to de Beauvoir, ultimately reality (de Beauvoir 1948: 156). For Halbwachs our memories are reconstructed under societal pressures—they conform to the strictures required of their deployment in any social setting. When it comes to fun these are many and various. They can be used to let people know the distance a person has travelled from one part of their life to another or they can be a claim to knowledge or legitimacy. For example, a middle-aged person may wish to demonstrate an understanding of young people and having fun and recall, 'I used to take lots of drugs at free parties in the 90s—I remember once getting so off my face that me and my friend ended up on a train. We were laughing so much we forgot that we didn't need to get a train and ended up in Yeovil.' This testimony can be manipulated to service whatever situation the holder of the memory wishes it to. Again, as per Halbwachs:

> Society from time to time obligates people not just to reproduce in thought previous events of their lives, but also to touch them up, to shorten them, or to complete them so that, however convinced we are that our memories are exact, we give them prestige that reality did not possess. (Halbwachs [1950] 1992: 51)

Whilst it is clearly the case that individuals have memories that are distinct to them, it is curious that they appear to be relatively coherent between people. If I recall moments of fun or levity, it is normally the case that others will be able to identify with that memory and recall similar incidents that inspired similar sentiments. For my fun to exist in memories, it needs to be understood by others as fun. This is part of the process of conditioning memories to fit with societal or group expectations—even when we are attempting to subvert expectations, by recounting experiences as fun that others might not recognise as fun, we tend to do so knowingly.

> What makes recent memories hang together is not that they are contiguous in time: it is rather that they are part of a totality of thoughts common to a group of people with whom we have a relation on the preceding day or days. To recall them is hence sufficient that we place ourselves in the perspective of this group, that we adopt its interests and follow the slant of its reflections. (Halbwachs [1950] 1992: 52)

This commonality, which is important for comprehension, does not look too distant from the Weberian concept of ideal types (Weber [1904] 1971: 63–7), but I think it is subtler than that. There is no requirement for common comprehension outside of the implications the recounting of memories has for identity. In terms of fun, it is important to know what people found fun and what they find fun now. As so much of the social distribution of narratives of fun is done through storytelling—as was suggested in the chapter on 'phenomenal fun'—the communication of stories of fun-making are important for determining what is considered fun and what is not. It is the communication of fun times or fun activities that then speak to the sort of collective memory phenomenon that was illustrated in the chapter on 'childhood and fun'. From the survey that was conducted for this book, the recurrent themes of fun in childhood for people that grew up in the UK was startling, and there was much less diversity than in the data on recent occasions of where adult respondents had fun. For a student of Halbwachs, this points to the observation that collective memories—the memories that we all hold in various forms but which bind us together—are socially constructed. The fun times that were reported in childhood are understood by others to be constitutive of a 'good' and perhaps, for those in Britain, 'British' childhood. It is easier to imagine that smaller groups have collective memories. Families, corporations, trades unions, friendship networks and even social classes have collective memories—as do whole societies, and these are often profoundly expressed through nationalist discourses.

From these groups, large and small, individuals draw on the collective constructions to reimagine their past. As I have suggested, it is not that our past is a pure invention; rather, that elements that fit with the collective memory are highlighted or amplified and those elements that do not fit or are not important are toned down or excluded. This is not a consciously strategic process, but happens without fuss. Memories are organised by us to make sense of the past in the present, and that present is sensitive to social pressures.

So, our individual memories are influenced by collective memories and these are socially constructed. Our individual memories are also organised by us but are no less individually meaningful as a result of these external and internal interferences. This is because memories are deployed to work for us. Memories of events that we have personally experienced are used to strengthen bonds between participants in any given group. Memories of fun times between friends are extremely important to maintaining many forms of friendship, particularly over time. As groups of people get older circumstances change, and in some instances people change. As an example, this is a common experience for those people lucky enough to go to university. As the years progress, former groups of friends drift apart, but when they get together, the glue that holds their friendship together are the stories from their university days—it is this that they all have in common and the memories get replayed and modified over the years to suit the changing circumstances of the individuals comprising the group.

When retelling stories of fun we are expecting others to acknowledge that our experiences are indeed fun and this confirms that our group—or people like us—understand that fun is had in this way. The telling of memories or stories as they become are also important for keeping events in the past alive. Lewis Coser suggests that 'it stands to reason that autobiographical memory tends to fade with time unless it is periodically reinforced through contact with persons with who one shared the experience with in the past' (Coser 1992: 24). Whilst memories have connections to actual events, sensations or whatever, the past is a social construction shaped by concerns of the present. The relationship between individual memory and the social mechanisms that exert force upon it is neatly summarised by Coser when he says 'memory needs continuous feeding from collective sources and is sustained by social and moral props' (Coser 1992: 34).

Fun, Recollection

The groups referred to by Halbwachs are fairly oblique in their constitution. It is sometimes difficult to know the scale and scope of the process of collective memory to which he refers. However, when it comes to collective fun the scale and scope is as large and wide as it is small and discrete. It seems to me that each society has a fairly clear idea of the sorts of things that are legitimately fun and those things that are not. It is interesting that this often involves the sorts of transgressions that elsewhere members of societies are expected to frown upon. Perhaps this is one of the important features of fun in that the subversive nature of it—celebrated and understood in one context or collective memory—is irritating or dangerous to another set of collective ideals celebrated elsewhere. For example, the regulation of fun at work (Chap. 5) where the sorts of fun made by workers stands in contrast to an ideal of good conduct of a worker or of the corporate aspirations of employers. It is also clear that people tend to think that fun can be atomised down to the individual level. As Will Self's protagonist in 'My Idea of Fun' illustrates, it is entirely reasonable to assume that there are some activities, sensations or whatever that would be experienced as fun for a very small number of people in any population.

Cultural Mediation of Fun

The embeddedness of particular narratives about what is fun and what isn't, how best to have fun and when to have fun are all artefacts of culture. In a similar way to Aries suggesting that childhood is understood between generations in different ways, the same can be said of fun. Unlike childhood, however, the fracture lines between what constitutes fun are not just intergenerational. They are also mediated by social class, gender, geography and all sorts of other variables that contribute to our experience of any given society. This cultural mediation highlights the complex relationship that we have with fun where social influences, identity, biography, circumstances and subjective phenomenal experiences of the world meet with our interpretations of the past—recent and distant—to produce orientations to present and future experiences of fun.

The cultural mediation of experiences of fun shares some features with humour, and in this instant, using humour by means of explanation is appropriate. As Gary Alan Fine notes:

> Most humor and laughter imply a social relationship, a connection between self and other. Just as one cannot tickle oneself, so, too, one can hardly tell oneself a joke or play a prank on oneself. A jocular event typically requires a minimum of two persons to succeed—or, for that matter, to fail. Although I shall not argue whether an event is not funny if there is no person there to observe it, any adequate understanding of the dynamics of humor must include a social analysis. (Fine 1983: 159)

Further to the idea that humour is a social activity, it is also the case that it can only be recognised as humour if the social group decides something is funny. As Mary Douglas notes:

> All jokes are expressive of the social situations in which they occur. The one social condition necessary for a joke to be enjoyed is that the social group in which it is received should develop the formal characteristics of a 'told' joke: that is, a dominant pattern of relations is challenged by another. (Douglas 1968: 366)

I do not want to interrogate humour in any depth, as too often 'funny' and 'fun' are seen as synonymous or mutually inclusive, which they are neither. However, it is interesting to note that the social or cultural embeddedness of both humour and fun rely to a large extent on understanding how these things are supposed to work in an iterative sense. The communication of both humour and fun relies on understanding what the collective memory of appropriate behaviour, response or way of communicating is. This is a learned process, one which involves immersion in a culture in such a way that fun is understood to consist of certain features, something is experienced which may or may not be fun, and is then replayed back as fun. This is not to say that people do not experience fun, but in recollection or casting back, fun is constructed and reconstructed in ways that are communicable to others. In this way cultures of social class, ethnicity, locality, age, fashion can be made distinct in the fun that they have because of the reiteration of culture through stories of fun. This is what people like us find fun. So the retelling of particular types of fun is important not just for identity but also for maintaining relationships in groups—and these groups can be tiny (this is what my friends and I like to do) or they can be enormous (this is what the British find fun).

Universalising Fun, Recollection and Identity

As with most subjective experiences, measuring them has an inevitable reductive impact. The tendency to imagine that those elements of life that contribute positively to well-being can be quantified or generalised is misguided. In the process of agglomeration, at some point culture is lost to features of fun or happiness that appear to reside in the present. Attempts in producing specific types of organised fun in workplaces or education seem doomed to fail, particularly in the light of what many people have said to me when I have asked them about fun at work, or fun in schools. Part of the problem is that popularly we understand that having fun is a positive affective response to current active situations, but as I am suggesting here, this is not an adequate description of how people relate to it. The status of fun is often applied retrospectively to things that have happened, and which are not necessarily understood as fun at the time. One obvious reason for this is that a key component in lots of fun is that the protagonist is distracted away from concentrating on anything but the experience itself. The naming of it as fun often happens after the event—either immediately after or in the retelling to another sometime later. A sensibility towards fun develops over time and involves our understanding of the nuances in our own identities—those aspect which are indicative of the sorts of people that we think we are, and as is widely recognised in sociology at least, these can be big, monolithic constructs like national identity to very small networked subcultures like groups of friends. Throughout the gradations of our identities, orientations and affective responses to phenomena develop, and keep developing, to produce a subjective orientation to something like fun that appears to be the preserve of the individual. This is a consequence of the multitudinal influences on identity that conspire to produce individuals.

An interesting finding from the chapter on fun in childhood was the relative uniformity in the responses of people when asked to remember occasions of fun in their past. This may on the surface appear to contradict what I have just said about generalising fun, but the point here is that this is not about experiencing fun in the moment, but communicating past fun in the present. The stories of adventure, freedom, holidays, family, being out of doors speak to us on a number of levels. As I suggested in the introduction, we establish a number of backdrops where we understand fun to have happened. These are then used as an ideal type mechanism for then communicating to others, not just fun that we have had, but also what sort of a childhood we wish to communicate to others, what sorts of families we come from and what sort of people we are that we understand certain activities as fun. The majority of the respondents in the survey were from the UK and the communication of fun from childhood speaks to a particularly British orientation to fun. That is not to say that people not from Britain would struggle to recognise the stories as fun, just that they are located and told in ways peculiar to the cultures from which they derive.

References

Bryant, F., Smart, C., & King, S. (2005). Using the past to enhance the present: Boosting happiness through positive reminiscence. *Journal of Happiness Studies, 6*, 227–260.

Collet-Sabe, J., & Tort, A. (2015). What do families of the 'professional and managerial' class educate their children for? The links between happiness and autonomy. *British Journal of Sociology of Education, 36*(2), 234–249.

Coser, L. (1992). Introduction. In M. Halbwachs (Ed.), *On collective memory*. Chicago: University of Chicago Press.

de Beauvoir, S. (1948). *Ethics of ambiguity*. New Jersey: Citadel Press.

Douglas, M. (1968). The social control of cognition: Some factors in joke perception. *Man, 3*(3), 361–376.

Einstein, G., Holland, L., McDaniel, M., & Guynn, M. (1992). Age-related deficits in prospective memory: The influence of task complexity. *Psychology and Aging, 7*(3), 471–478.

Fine, G. A. (1983). Sociological approaches to the study of humor. In P. McGhee & J. Goldstein (Eds.), *The handbook of humor research*. New York: Springer.

Halbwachs, M. ([1950] 1992). On collective memory. Chicago: University of Chicago Press.

Mather, M., & Carstensen, L. (2005). Aging and motivated cognition: The positivity effect in attention and memory. *Trends in Cognitive Sciences, 9*(10), 496–502.

Phillips, D. (1969). Social class, social participation, and happiness: A consideration of interaction opportunities and investment. *The Sociological Quarterly, 10*(1), 3–21.

Schlagman, S., Schulz, J., & Kvavilashvili, L. (2006). A content analysis of involuntary autobiographical memories: Examining the positivity effect in old age. *Memory, 14*(2), 161–175.

Weber, M. ([1904] 1971). The ideal type. In Thompson, K. & Tunstall, J. (1971) *Sociological perspectives*. Harmondsworth: Pelican.

8

Conclusions

Fun is a complex thing. It is experienced in the moment but is also a discourse, applied retrospectively. It is a part of the glue that binds together social groups and also informs individuals' identity. It is something that is unruly and spontaneous but has recently become part of a movement towards organised forms. It is a battleground in schools and work between the will of students or workers to be autonomous and carefree against the wishes of forces of control and production. It is important and frivolous. Our experience of it is ours alone yet it has to resonate with others in order to be recognised as fun. It is related to pleasure and happiness but is distinct from both. This book has not sought to simplify this complexity but rather to acknowledge, and to a certain extent, celebrate it. Whilst I have presented a model of fun (Chap. 2), this is just a suggestion of how to discern fun from other affective domains. I have not intended to be overly reductionist in describing or explaining fun. Like Blythe and Hassenzahl, I see fun as sitting along continua in the relationship it has with its constituent components. Rather than presenting absolutes it is more sensible to talk about degrees, when characterising where an experience of fun sits in relation to, for example, commitment. The other purpose of this book is to present everyday accounts of fun.

The data represented here are the thoughts of people that had not spent much time hitherto wondering what their fun consisted of. For many it was an interesting and surprising exercise. I received messages and had conversations with lots of people saying that they had spent a long time after being asked the questions in the survey, pondering quite how and when they had fun. It sparked a great number of conversations between people and for me that is a positive consequence of having initiated this particular branch of a sociology of fun.

Fun, Happiness and Pleasure

The distinctions between fun, happiness and pleasure—related phenomena—are clear when experiences or 'exciting goings on' (Blythe and Hassenzahl 2004: 92) are considered in relation to the model presented in Chap. 2 and whilst nobody that I have spoken to about fun over the last few years will have seen that model, many of the core items were picked up by people that I surveyed. Having said that, it was clear that many people had not previously considered the distinctiveness of fun from, for example, well-being, pleasure or happiness. When asked, people did attempt to explain differences whilst still acknowledging interrelatedness; this is despite many struggling to express exactly what they meant. Most people picked out the idea that fun was more active than pleasure or happiness. People said things like 'for me fun usually means when I am doing something that I enjoy and happiness and pleasure are the feelings I get from having fun' (F19, Student). For this person 'doing something' was a place where they could draw a distinction between their experiences of fun, pleasure and happiness. Another said:

> Fun is about play for me, about shedding worries or responsibilities. Happiness is a state of being, not necessarily tied to an action, like fun is (unless you count sitting and thinking as an action). Pleasure and fun are harder for me to separate, but pleasure is more about satisfying a need or a want than playing. (T22, Student)

Associated with being active was also the idea of carefree times or abandon as well as the invocation of activity as a defining characteristic in relation to happiness or pleasure. One person summed this up nicely and said, 'Fun almost seems like the action, whereas happiness is seen as a feeling' (F20, Student). Temporality will be discussed in more detail a little later, but for those responding to the survey this was another key feature of fun as opposed to pleasure or happiness. A student from France said, 'Happiness is more extended over a longer period, it's also deeper, not necessarily attached to lightheartedness' (F26, Student). A teacher summed it up neatly suggesting, 'Fun is in passing. Happiness is more lasting. Pleasure is a mixture of both' (F57, Teacher). Some thought about where the temporality resides in the different affective states—if their relationships to it are different. One person said:

> I think fun is more experience based, it is much more of 'the moment' than happiness or pleasure. I think it's transitory, and 'instances' of fun can be related to others easily. Whereas happiness tends to define a state of mind, and pleasure has a connotation of commodification and a purchased experience. (M32, Student)

For this person the resonance of time in happiness is that it is much more related to a state of mind that is not necessarily bound by immediate experiences. A person that worked on a checkout at a supermarket drew the active and the temporal together:

> Happiness is long term and pleasure seems like a physical experience. Fun is a short term experience that combines the physicality of pleasure, and the long term memory of happiness. (F21, Shop worker)

Another element that came from the question about the difference between fun, pleasure and happiness was the social element of fun, as opposed to pleasure or happiness with one person summarising what many said, 'For me, fun involves doing pleasurable or happy stuff with other people. I can be happy when I'm alone but I can't have fun on my own' (F45, Senior research officer). Several people also mentioned the idea of both the spontaneity and the unpredictability of fun with one person saying, 'I feel that happiness/pleasure is like being wrapped in a warm blanket, you know the emotion, you know why you feel this way whereas with fun you don't know how it will end or how far it will go' (F41, P16 Vocational learning manager).

As I have said, when asked everybody that I have spoken to acknowledges that fun is different to pleasure and happiness. This is not understood to be a semantic difference and the terms are deployed in specific contexts to describe specific things. It is interesting though that relatively few people had a ready answer to what the distinctions between these phenomena are. The fact that we are unused to thinking too deeply about what fun consists of contributes to not just its marginal status as something to be taken seriously,[1] but also makes it relatively easy to unreflexively fold fun into concepts deemed to be more important—happiness, well-being, for example—or position fun as an experience that can be sidelined in favour of things that we already acknowledge as being important. To return to where this book started, it is still a source of bemusement to me that fun is not part of any well-being survey. Whilst I would be critical of its appearance as something that is difficult to quantify, I would have assumed that somebody might have recognised it as an important factor in what makes people feel good about life. Another contributing factor to the marginalisation of fun is its relationship to temporality. The lack of temporal resonance of fun—the idea that it is fleeting simply amplifies the view of it as frivolous and without depth. As has been pointed out throughout the previous chapters, one of the greatest dichotomies of fun is that it is defined partly through its lack of seriousness—and a lack of seriousness, a carefree outlook or alleviation from current concerns or anxieties is important for our happiness. I would go as far as suggesting that fun is essential for a fulfilling life. The dichotomy that something frivolous and trivial is so important is at the heart of this endeavour—and it is partly this contradiction that has left fun outside of the consideration of sociology.

The broader relative marginality of fun also means that it can be cajoled and bullied into discrete places and times throughout our schooling and into our working lives. We are trained to understand fun as trivial or frivolous in certain settings, thus making it easier to control. A key aspect of some forms of fun is deviation from norms. Where Becker's 'infraction of some agreed upon rule' (Becker 1963: 8) establishes the grounds

---

[1] I am aware that this sounds like a contradiction in terms.

for transgressive fun workplaces and schools are keen to inhibit this sort of fun as much as possible. They are institutionally invested in policing rules. However, in much the way described by Illich with schooling and Gorz with work, I would advocate a much freer attitude to the ways in which time and space are controlled. Throughout the data that I have gathered regarding work and fun, it is clear that many people spend a lot of time in environments where their fun is tightly controlled through the routines of the working day. People described chatting as fun in workplaces where talk in productive time was controlled or discouraged. The overwhelming sense from these data is that work is not a lot of fun. An important point to emerge is that the sorts of ways of describing fun—or its absence—at work today is very similar to descriptions as far back as the 1940s and 1950s. Whilst forms of work have changed a great deal in the last 70 years, our responses to being at work appear relatively unaltered in relation to fun at any rate.

Fun as a Social Activity

A defining characteristic of fun is that it is social—and this contrasts with descriptions of it in naturalistic terms (see Vanderschuren 2010). Whilst it may well be the case that there are neurological processes that support fun-having, the social element is what makes an experience, activity or moment fun. It is had with others, in anticipation of being with others or in relation to absent others. Throughout the survey, time and again, people explained that fun was had with, and in relation to, other people. It serves a dual purpose in that it establishes and maintains bonds between people and, in a reflexive sense, informs identity. What we do for fun and who we have fun with say much about who we are.

The primacy of social interaction and identity in having fun presents problems when it comes to organised or packaged fun. The idea that we experience events or happenings in similar ways, because they are designed to be fun, cannot account for the individualised ways in which social interaction occurs. Further, our reaction to social circumstances is contextual—it does not matter how much a person enjoys going bowling; if they do not like their work colleagues and are made to go to the local bowling alley for a team building event, they will not find it fun.

Acknowledging that fun is a social phenomenon distances it from the idea that activities are in and of themselves fun. A good example is demonstrated through literature on the benefits of making sport fun for schoolchildren (e.g., Portman 1995; O'Reilly et al. 2001; Macphail et al. 2008; Visek et al. 2015). Many articles discuss the difficulty of engaging young people in physical activity, and a default response is to suggest that the solution is to make it fun. Discussion of quite how to do this is limited to attempting to appeal to young peoples' sense of playfulness. However, this approach only addresses part of the issue. Until the primacy of social relations in fun is taken into account, the assumption that sport can become in and of itself fun will not work. Fun happens because of the context within which specific social relations occur. It is for this reason that 'organised', encouraged or forced fun will forever be faced with dread by participants, especially if social relationships are not put at the heart of activities assumed to be fun. Even then organisers of fun events face an uphill battle to foster fun when autonomy and transgression are often parts of our translation of experiences or happenings as fun. Following Gorz's ideas about subjection, manufactured fun is an attempt to control social interactions within environments where adherence to rules and control are privileged or important. When it comes to school and work the control of fun and a relationship to productivity is clear. The necessity to inculcate a population with the idea that fun is important but only in the right time and place becomes apparent when data about experiences of work is examined. It is in the interests of employers that they control how employees use time. The idea that something as non-productive as fun might happen in productive time is the antithesis of the logic of capitalist employment practice, and school is where we compartmentalise fun into the routines that then are reflected in work. Given the etymology of the word fun and the association with transgressing rules, it is no surprise that the fun that individuals create and are involved in stands at odds with the intentions or aspirations of the school or the workplace. It explains why we are so often at odds with formalised rules—creative, autonomous fun can only be had in opposition to the intentions of institutional control of time and behaviour.

In childhood the positive experiences manifest in relationships with others are clear. In particular, family provides a locus for experiences of fun, but also friends are important. Alongside these relationships are the backdrops mentioned in the Introduction. The outdoors, holidays and games are sites where fun happens. In early adulthood our dependence on family weakens and friends become more prominent in how we experience fun, and this continues until, for those that have them, children arrive and there is a retrenchment into narratives of fun as mediated through family.

Temporality

There are particular aspects of temporality that are important to understanding fun. In terms of experiences we tend to be able to identify when fun starts and when it stops. It does not resonate through time—backwards and forwards—in the way that pleasure but particularly happiness does. This process of understanding fun as being the preserve of discrete moments starts in childhood. Glenn et al. suggest the children that they studied were quite clear in their demarcation of time in relation to fun and play. In fact, it was so clear that they suggest that when the fun stopped the play stopped (Glenn et al. 2012: 190). As this interpretation is so clearly associated with activities, it is easy to discern the times between which fun is being had. As was illustrated in data presented in this book, people themselves understand that fun has a special and overt relationship to time. Of course this is not to say that people cannot identify discrete periods of happiness or pleasure, but this clarity of periods of time is not understood as a core, defining characteristic of either happiness or pleasure—where it is with fun.

Whilst this appears relatively straightforward there is also a relationship to reconstruction and remembering that involves temporality, and an interesting intersection with identity. As has been suggested, fun often involves engrossment in it, and as a consequence, distraction away from other things—like analysing what sort of a time you are having. We rarely think 'this is fun', or ask ourselves the question 'is this fun?' What does happen is that we apply the status of fun to periods of time after the event. This is not to suggest that the experience was not fun, simply that we could not identify it as such at the time, as that would involve a process that would alter the distracted state on which the fun relies. It is often in the retelling of an experience that fun is applied as a descriptor for it. This performs several functions. The first is that it establishes a common ground for understanding experiences. The naturalistic tendency—to imagine that because we are human we experience things similarly—is compounded by the establishment of discourses that appear to describe uniformly understood phenomena. This is particularly true of fun. The fact that people that I spoke to generally struggled to describe what fun is but at the same time had no trouble describing things unproblematically, as fun suggests that there is an assumption that we mean the same thing when we say it. Also, that there was relatively little variance in the stories that were provided to describe fun in childhood, and fun in adulthood makes it seem as though we have a clear idea of what fun consists of and we all experience it in similar ways. This may also be true to an extent, but this is because of the cultural embeddedness of discourses of fun. We iterate our fun in ways that make sense to other people—fun is interactional and requires affirmation from others for the necessary social conditions for it to be satisfied. Often, I suspect, in the telling of times of fun, fun is had. In the reconstituting of positive times there is a secondary fun that comes in reminiscence. The lack of diversity of stories of fun from childhood in my survey speaks not just to the types of fun we actually have, but also how ideal types of childhood and relationships with others are understood and replayed. In a sense we do to the past what Judith Butler suggests we do to the body when becoming gendered (Butler 1990)—but rather than a body that is prey to repeated stylisation, it is the past. Halbwachs explicitly draws our attention to how this process perpetuates identity (Halbwachs 1992: 47); through this consistent reiteration of the past we maintain our sense of who we think we are and where we have come from.

Commitment, Responsibility and Anticipation

In order for fun to take place commitment and responsibility must be temporarily suspended. Commitment involves 'being absorbed or committed to an activity' and 'involves acceptance of assumptions and rules surrounding that activity'. It is reasonable to assume that we can be committed to an activity that we also experience as fun; however, the idea of commitment for Blythe and Hassenzahl and, for that matter, me involves a task, a concern or period of 'not fun time' from which we become distracted. It involves an orientation to task or experience that is then temporarily suspended during the times at which we have fun. Similarly, we must be temporarily alleviated from present concerns or anxieties. During fun attention is directed away from responsibility towards a more carefree attitude—however short-lived that may be. It is not necessarily the case that fun is defined through irresponsibility but that responsibility is not a concern during periods of fun. Anticipation is more complex than commitment or responsibility. In the moment, anticipation of what will or ought to happen next is suspended. Several people in the survey expressed the excitement of unpredictability in fun. At the same time, there is often an assumption that a situation that has been experienced as fun will be fun once more. We can recognise a situation, or even a sensation, and then anticipate that it will be fun not because of a prediction of what will happen but because of an identification with something that has *already* happened—a fun experience in the past. In this way, retrospection works with anticipation to create an openness to a situation as fun.

So What...?

There are many things that have not been addressed in this book. There are questions of gender, social class, ethnicity, cross-cultural comparison, for example, that have not been accounted for here. There is clearly more to be said about the fluidity of definition and context dependency of experiences with regard to fun. However, as was stated at the beginning of the book, this is very much a starting point for further discussion about the nature and importance of fun, about what sorts of aspects of fun we are willing to cede to others and the extent to which we choose to celebrate or repress the more transgressive elements of our fun. Here I have presented a model for understanding experiences as fun, but this is not intended to suggest that other things that do not seem to fit neatly into the schema are not fun. Whilst I think that there are strong discourses that guide what most people understand as being fun—and I think that the model of fun is useful to understanding distinctions between phenomena—there is always the deviant and autonomous fun that is owned by the interactants, and that does not necessarily fit neatly into models. As I have used Blythe and Hassenzahl as a building block, I hope subsequent writers about fun will do the same with this book.

Fun is very important. It provides levity in the face of boredom or sadness. It is essential for feeling good. It fuels families and friendships, identities and happiness. It is something to be nurtured and cherished, enhanced, encouraged, recognised and celebrated. We will experience it in our own ways but always have it with others, and as long as there are rules, there will be people playfully breaking them, having fun.

References

Becker, H. (1963). *Outsiders*. New York: Free Press.

Blythe, M., & Hassenzahl, M. (2004). The semantics of fun: Differentiating enjoyable experiences. In M. Blythe, K. Overbeeke, A. Monk, & P. Wright (Eds.), *Funology: From usability to enjoyment*. London: Kluwer.

Butler, J. (1990). *Gender trouble*. London: Routledge.

Glenn, N., Knight, C., Holt, N., & Spence, J. (2012). Meanings of play among children. *Childhood, 20*(2), 185–199.

Halbwachs, M. ([1950] 1992). On collective memory. Chicago: University of Chicago Press.

MacPhail, A., Gorely, T., Kirk, D., & Kinchin, G. (2008). Exploring the meaning of fun in physical education the sport education. *Research Quarterly for Exercise and Sport, 79*(3), 344–356.

O'Reilly, E., Tompkins, J., & Gallant, M. (2001). 'They ought to enjoy physical activity you know?' Struggling with fun in physical education. *Sport Education and Society, 6*(2), 211–221.

Portman, P. (1995). Who is having fun in physical education classes? Experiences of sixth grade students in elementary and middle schools. *Journal of Teaching in Physical Education, 14*, 445–453.

Vanderschuren, L. (2010). How the brain makes play fun. *American Journal of Play Winter, 2010*, 315–337.

Visek, A., Achrati, S., Manning, H., McDonnell, K., Harris, B., & di Pietro, L. (2015). The fun integration theory: Towards sustaining youth and adolescents sports participation. *Journal of Physical Activity and Health, 12*(3), 424–433.

Bibliography

Austen, J. (1992). *Pride and prejudice*. London: Penguin.
Baldry, C., & Hallier, J. (2009). Welcome to the house of fun: Work space and social identity. *Economic and Industrial Democracy, 31*(1), 150–172.
Ballas, D. (2010). Geographical modelling of happiness and wellbeing. In J. Stillwell, P. Norman, C. Thomas, & P. Surridge (Eds.), *Spatial and social disparities: Understanding population trends and processes* (Vol. 2). London/New York: Springer.
Butsch, R. (1990a). Introduction: Leisure and hegemony in America. In R. Butsch (Ed.), *For fun and profit: The transformation of leisure into consumption*. Philadelphia: Temple University Press.
Butsch, R. (1990b). *For fun and profit: The transformation of leisure into consumption*. Philadelphia: Temple University Press.
Chan, C. (2010). Does workplace fun matter? Developing a useable typology of workplace fun in qualitative study. *International Journal of Hospitality Management, 29*, 720–728.
Cox, R. (1996). *Shaping childhood: Themes of uncertainty in the history of adult-child relationships*. London/New York: Routledge.
de Beauvoir, S. (1974[1949]). *The second sex*. New York: Vintage.
Erickson, M. (2010). Efficiency and effort revisited. In M. Erickson & C. Turner (Eds.), *The sociology of Wilhelm Baldamus*. Farnham: Ashgate.

Fleming, P., & Sturdy, A. (2009). "Just be yourself!" Towards neo-normative control in organisations? *Employee Relations, 31*(6), 569–583.

Self, W. (1993). *My idea of fun*. London: Bloomsbury.

Smith, D. B. (1980). *Inside the great house: Planter family life in eighteenth century Chesapeake society*. Ithaca: Cornell University Press.

Sutton, R. (2001). *Weird ideas that work: 11 ½ ways to promote, manage and sustain innovation*. New York: Penguin.

Veblen, T. (2007 [1899]). *Theory of the leisure class*. Oxford: Oxford University Press.

Wilson, W. (2012). *Nature and young children: Encouraging creative play and learning in natural environments*. Abingdon: Routledge.

Index

A
Absorbtion, 36–37, 60–64, 195
Adolescence, 22, 50, 83, 86–92
Adults/Adulthood, 1, 8, 16, 22, 47–49, 53–54, 57–64, 83–120, 187–189
Adventure, 39, 60–64, 195
Aesthetics, 37–38, 172h
Affect, 8, 12, 27, 33, 39, 59, 155, 160, 163–164, 168, 194
Alcohol, 18, 84, 94, 107–109, 112, 119–120
Animals, 54, 58, 70–71, 107
Anticipation, 37, 42, 151, 186, 201, 204–206
Aries, P., 50–51, 92, 192
Autonomy, 131, 134, 146, 202

B
Backdrops, 17–21, 195, 203
Baldamus, G., 122, 131–132, 136, 148
Banter, 100, 105, 135–139, 148–150
Beach, 11, 18, 61, 64–65, 69–76, 79, 84, 101, 105
Becker, H., 13, 41, 87–89, 119, 122, 200–201
Being-in-the-moment, 5, 17–18, 42, 44–45, 85, 97, 110, 122–123, 156–161, 163–172, 175–181, 205
Biology, 51, 54, 57–58
Blythe, M. and Hassenzahl, M., 6–7, 15–17, 28–29, 35–45, 56, 62, 66, 93, 115, 150, 167, 187, 197–198, 205–206
Bodies, 157, 161, 164, 170, 181
Boredom, 83, 122, 132, 145, 151, 206
Branson, R., 126, 134

C

Cadbury's, 124–125, 128, 145
Chatting, 83, 105–108, 136–139, 145, 149
Childish, 14, 76, 83, 86–87, 92, 94, 115–116, 143, 184, 188
Children, 7, 11, 15, 49–65, 69–80, 83–95, 113–116, 144, 187
Collective Memory, 190–193
Commitment, 17, 37–42, 45, 56, 87, 93, 115, 151, 204–205
Computer games, 35, 98
Computers, 27, 35, 57, 70, 79, 150
Consumption, 7, 31
Contexts, 3, 7, 9, 12–18, 33, 35–36, 43, 50–51, 55, 58, 83, 86–87, 119–120, 155, 162–165, 179, 189, 200–202, 205
Conversation, 105, 146, 157
Cornwall, 29
Creativity, 78, 92, 119, 132, 138–129, 151–152, 202
Culture, 7, 23, 29, 38, 130, 133–134, 193–195
Cycling, 63, 105, 156, 183

D

Dancing, 35, 44, 64, 85, 95, 108, 178
de Beauvoir, S., 160, 189
Disinhibition, 94–95, 100, 119, 156, 179
Distraction, 8, 30, 36–37, 44–45, 118, 121–123, 128, 132, 135–137, 145, 150–152, 164–166, 175, 177–180, 194, 203–204
Dualism, 55–56

E

Economics, 2, 4, 9, 35, 50, 124, 129–130
Education, 2–3, 15–17, 51, 53, 78, 89, 161, 194
Embodiment, 22, 32, 155–163, 166, 170–181
Emotion, 27–28, 131–133, 142, 176–177, 180–181, 185, 199
Emotional Labour, 131, 142
Enjoyment, 7–8, 31–39, 45–46, 92–94
Euphoria, 44, 85, 161, 172, 174–175, 178, 180

F

Family, 1–3, 14–15, 50–51, 60, 64–69, 72, 99–103, 119, 186–187, 189, 202–203
Feelings, 6, 56, 85, 132, 156, 163–200
Festivals, 19, 85, 112
Flow, 159, 161–162
Food, 117
Forgetting, 161, 167, 175
Freedom, 8, 12, 31–33, 42, 50, 52, 56, 63–64, 73, 85, 102, 134, 149–150, 156, 164–168, 174, 179, 197–198, 205
Friends, 2, 11–12, 15–16, 33, 62–64, 67–68, 72–79, 84, 96–113, 116–119, 142, 170, 187, 190–191, 203, 206
Frivolity, 5, 8, 10, 15, 22–23, 30–31, 54, 58, 93, 156, 197, 200
Fun Morality, 3, 10, 80, 88, 134, 185

G

Games, 38, 56–58, 60–62, 68, 73–77, 113, 129, 143–145, 149, 187, 203
Gender, 19, 43, 45, 151, 204–205
Gigs, 110–112
Google, 124, 126, 128, 133–135
Gorz, A., 126, 129, 134, 146, 201–202
Grandchildren, 65, 87, 94, 100

H

Halbwachs, M., 186–192, 204
Happiness, 1–5, 7, 9–10, 19–24, 27–30, 32–41, 43, 49, 59, 66, 90, 115, 125, 127, 130–133, 147, 155, 159–166, 170–171, 176–180, 187, 197–200, 203, 206
Holidays, 11, 15, 30, 60–66, 68–72, 85, 99, 104, 109–110, 119, 195, 203
Home, 41, 64, 76, 110, 130
Human, 12, 28, 34, 126, 159, 161, 172, 204
Humour, 11–12, 129–130, 138–142

I

Identity, 10–11, 19, 29, 33, 43, 45, 79, 84, 104, 123, 134, 151, 161, 184–195, 197, 201, 203–204
Ideology, 12, 34
Illich, I., 48, 79, 201
Inequality, 12
Innocence, 83, 92, 169
Innocent Drinks, 124, 126, 128, 135

J

Jokes, 65, 110, 135, 139–143, 150, 171, 193
Joking, 35, 97, 136–140
Joy, 28, 38, 78–79, 92, 104, 121, 130, 163, 171, 173–174, 176–177, 180, 186

L

Laughter, 6–7, 18, 48, 59, 64–65, 67, 76, 84–85, 100–101, 105–108, 110, 112, 116, 119, 124, 127–128, 136–141, 147–148, 166, 171–175, 179, 189
Learning, 15, 17, 47–49, 54, 65, 69, 90, 92
Leisure, 1, 3, 6–8, 16–18, 22, 29, 31
Leisure Studies, 1, 27, 29, 31
Life Course, 18, 86–88, 93, 103, 105, 113

M

Management, 123, 126, 128, 133, 140, 149, 152
Managers, 14, 124, 127, 133, 135, 140
Memory, 19, 22, 37, 72, 184, 186–194
Mental Health, 3–4, 10, 119, 122, 130
Merleau-Ponty, M., 104, 157–158
Money, 69, 101, 121
Mood, 14, 85, 95, 112, 133, 141
Morality, 10–11, 45, 80, 88, 134, 185
Music, 19, 35, 99, 103, 106, 110–112, 140, 187

N

Nature, 60, 63, 67, 70–76, 79, 99, 103–104, 203
Naughtiness, 61–63, 79, 110, 118, 134, 140–143, 150, 173, 187
Norms, 36, 89, 93–94, 127, 150–151, 188, 200

O

Organic fun, 79, 113, 126–130
Organised fun, 14–49, 79, 125–130, 143, 152, 194, 197, 201–202
Outdoors, 60, 63, 67, 70–76, 79, 99, 104–105, 119, 203

P

Packaged fun, 126–127, 130, 143, 201
Parents, 15, 18, 50, 62–67, 87, 94–95, 188
Parks, 8, 70, 72–73, 76, 79
Pedagogy, 15, 21, 47, 49, 59, 78, 90, 92
Phenomenology, 22, 33, 155–182
Philosophy, 2, 90, 128, 133
Physical Health, 9, 114–115, 125
Piaget, J., 52–55
Play, 11, 15, 41, 47–69, 72–79, 90, 92, 101–102, 105, 113, 116, 124, 128–131, 143–145, 149, 188, 198, 203
Pleasure, 5, 7, 22, 29, 31–34, 36–43, 49–50, 93–94, 147, 162–163, 168–169, 197–200, 203
Podilchak, W., 11–12, 27, 29, 31–34, 44–45, 110, 179

Power, 3, 11–12, 24, 29, 31–32, 34, 45, 48, 88, 110, 122, 141, 143, 179
Productivity, 6, 22, 41, 50, 57, 95, 121, 124–133, 145, 150–151, 201–202
Progression, 17, 37–38
Psychology, 29, 31, 37, 53–56, 130, 161
Pubs, 43, 84, 96, 103, 107–108, 111

R

Reconstruction, 183, 186–191, 203
Relevance, 36, 38
Reminiscence, 98, 184–185
Repetition, 16, 37–38, 66, 100
Resistance, 6, 19–20
Responsibilities/Responsibility, 30, 42, 45, 83–85, 88, 93, 119–120
Roy, D., 3, 9, 29, 31, 41, 115, 122, 130, 150
Rules, 15, 23, 38, 41, 47, 49, 56, 67, 92, 97, 115–116, 119, 140–143, 179, 201, 203–204, 206

S

Schema of fun, 39–40, 45, 147, 152, 172, 205
School, 15–16, 47–51, 54, 69, 78–79, 90–92, 197, 200–202
Sea/Seaside, 18, 65–72, 84, 112–114
Semantics, 5, 156, 181
Seriousness, 6, 12, 16, 30, 34, 37, 48, 57, 78, 93, 166, 169–170, 188, 200
Sex, 17, 31, 35, 102, 178

Situatedness, 32
Situational adjustment, 87–90
Smiling, 85, 164–166, 171–174, 176, 179
Social class, 6, 8–10, 20, 29–30, 43, 51, 79–80, 118, 120, 187, 191–192, 199, 205
Social experiences, 1, 5–6, 13, 17–24, 27–28, 34, 36, 44–47, 50, 56, 70, 101, 103, 120, 157–160, 164, 172–173, 179–181, 185, 191–194, 199, 201–206
Socialisation, 203
Social media, 11
Space, 7–8, 15, 18, 47–48, 63, 70, 73–74, 95, 112, 119, 150–151, 201
Spectacle, 37–38
Sport, 7–8, 57, 59, 75–77, 79, 93, 114, 125, 202
Subjectivity, 156
Subversion, 6, 9, 15, 90, 127, 129, 135, 138, 140–143, 149–150, 152, 192
Success, 2, 89, 146–147

T

Talking, 3, 31, 33, 35, 58, 97, 105–107, 119, 136–140
Temporality, 23, 32, 41, 45, 66, 156, 165, 172, 199
Time, 14–18, 28, 41–43, 47, 79, 89–90, 112, 119, 145–151, 165–167, 175, 194, 201–205
Traction, 48, 131–132, 147
Transcendence, 167–168

Transgressive, 6, 14, 22–23, 37–39, 41–43, 48, 56, 61–62, 79, 95, 115, 119, 142, 205
Triviality, 6, 33, 36–39, 66, 170, 200

U

Unselfconscious, 54, 165

V

Veblen, T., 16
Vygotsky, L., 52, 54–55, 58

W

Water, 1, 18, 60, 65, 70, 72–75, 84, 105, 109
  Pools, 74–75, 77, 100, 125
  Rain, 62
  Rivers, 62, 75, 107
Wealth, 2, 89
Weather, 64, 73–74, 76, 105
Weber, M., 44, 180, 190
Wellbeing, 4–5, 91
Well being index, 4–5
Wolfenstein, M., 10–11, 27, 29–31, 44–45, 49, 54, 79, 86, 134, 160
Work, 3–4, 6, 13–15, 30, 52, 95, 121–152, 192, 194, 201
Work-life balance, 14, 121, 125, 130–135, 160
Work Spaces, 128–130

Y

Yahoo, 124, 126, 128, 135
Youth, 8, 29, 50, 86, 118

The manufacturer's authorised representative in the EU is Springer Nature Customer Service Centre GmbH, Europaplatz 3, 69115 Heidelberg, Germany. If you have any concerns regarding our products, please contact ProductSafety@springernature.com

Printed and bound by CPI Group (UK) Ltd, Croydon, CR0 4YY

23/03/2026

02076459-0001